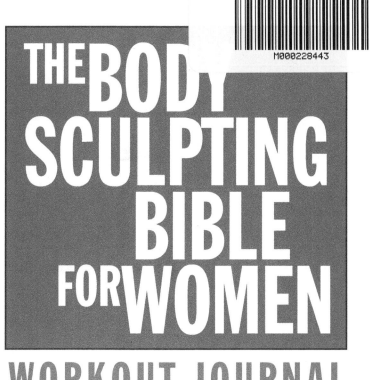

THE BODY SCULPTING BIBLE FOR WOMEN

WORKOUT JOURNAL

JAMES VILLEPIGUE
HUGO A. RIVERA

))) hatherleigh

Hatherleigh Press is committed to preserving and protecting the natural resources of the earth. Environmentally responsible and sustainable practices are embraced within the company's mission statement.

Visit us at www.hatherleighpress.com and register online for free offers, discounts, special events, and more.

The Body Sculpting Bible for Women Workout Journal
Text copyright © 2014 James Villepigue and Hugo Rivera

Library of Congress Cataloging-in-Publication Data is available upon request.
ISBN: 978-1-57826-524-4

Cover and Interior Design by Heather Magnan

Printed in the United States
10 9 8 7 6 5 4 3 2

Contents

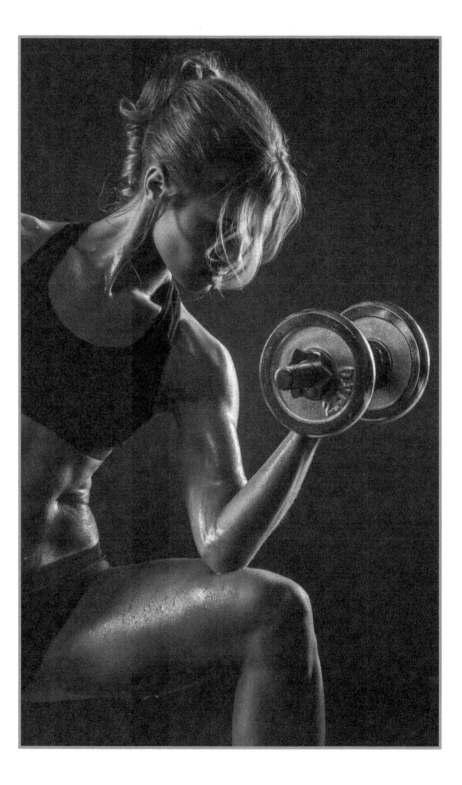

Introduction

INTRODUCTION

We've all imagined our "perfect" body and envisioned how great we would feel if we could just achieve that lofty goal. *The Body Sculpting Bible for Women Workout Journal* provides all of the tools you need to keep you motivated and keep your training workout on track so that your perfect body can become a reality!

Along with some dedication and hard work on your part, this journal will help you plan your regimen and measure your progress effectively. In the following pages, you will find lots of fitness tips, charts, and workout plans, along with daily nutrition and exercise logs to make it even easier to build muscle faster.

Keep *The Body Sculpting Bible for Women Workout Journal* in your gym bag and carry it with you throughout the day to log your nutrition and exercise. With this handy guide, you can finally take the guesswork out of your workout regimen so that you can focus on achieving your fitness goals.

For even more amazing results, pair this journal with any of the books in the *Body Sculpting Bible* series. Any of the *Body Sculpting Bible* workouts make the perfect companion to this journal and along with the workout plans in Body Sculpting Workouts (page 51), we give you suggestions for additional workouts within the *Body Sculpting Bible* series.

This journal has been designed based on invaluable expertise from two of bodybuilding's foremost authorities, James Villepigue and Hugo Rivera. We invite you to follow along on this journey, learn from the guidance provided in these pages, and finally achieve those amazing fitness results you never thought possible!

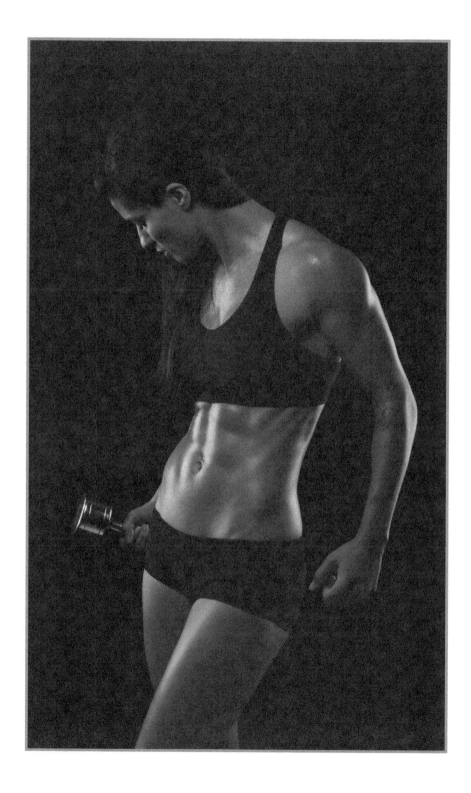

Part 1:
The Body Sculpting Program

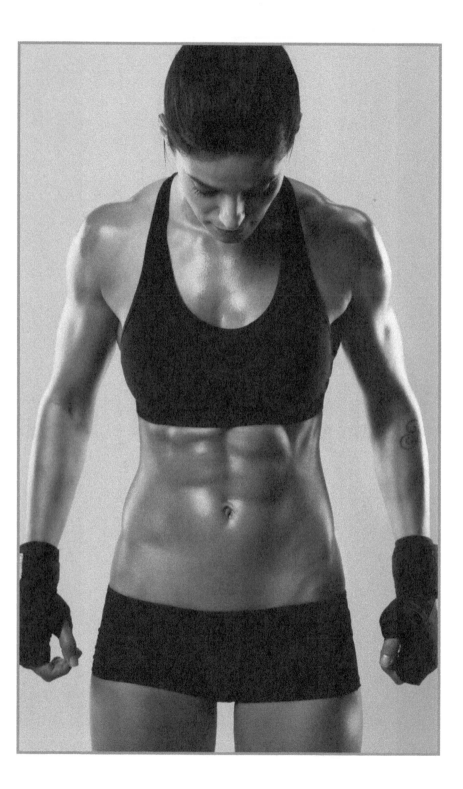

What is the 14-Day Body Sculpting Program?

THE SOLUTION TO FAT LOSS AND TONING

The 14-Day Body Sculpting Program is a system that takes a safe and holistic approach to fat loss and muscle toning that enables you to reach your goals in the minimum amount of time.

What is so unique about 14 days? Fourteen days is typically the amount of time that it takes to get used to a new habit. Also, 14 days is the amount of time that it takes the body to start getting used to a new training and nutrition scheme. Now, while it is good for us to get used to a new habit (like waking up early in the morning to work out), it is not good for the body to get used to our workout and nutrition program. The reason for that is because once the body adjusts to your workout routine and your current intake of calories, results will cease to come! So in other words, while you will still be working out in earnest and dieting, your body will remain at the same body fat percentage and your muscles will not change any further. This is why after you start a new exercise and nutrition program, you stop getting results after a few weeks.

Why does this happen? The reason for this is because the body likes to remain in a state of homeostasis (balance). In other words, our bodies like to remain the same way that they currently are. So when you start reducing calories in order to lose fat, your body goes ahead and starts losing fat. That is until it reduces its metabolism so that fat loss comes to a standstill. You see, our pre-historic ancestors sometimes would go through periods of famine and only the fat that their bodies had would keep them alive. Because of this, the body adapted to conserve energy (in the form of fat) in order to always be prepared for periods of low food consumption.

Now, what about muscle? Same thing here. When you start a weight training program, muscle tone comes quickly. However after a period of time of using the same routine the body learns to stay at the same fitness level. It does this in order to conserve energy as the more muscle you have, the more calories you burn. Not a good thing for our pre-historic ancestors to burn a lot of calories when no food was available. Therefore, the body is always attempting to get by with as little muscle as possible.

So how does the 14-Day Body Sculpting Program solve these problems? Because this system:

- Changes the parameters (sets, reps, and rest in between sets) of weight training routines every 14 days in a logical and periodized manner to ensure maximum workout efficiency (more on this later)
- Adjusts the duration of cardiovascular activities every 14 days
- Varies caloric intake every 14 days.

THE WEIGHT LOSS OBSESSION

First we ask you to stop obsessing about your bodyweight. Instead, focus on your bodily measurements, fat composition, and the way you look in the mirror. Why? Because weight cannot give you a true indication of how much fat you are carrying. Bodyweight is a combination of the weight of all of your bone structure, organs, muscles, water, and fat. Therefore, if you lose five pounds in one week, how can you be assured that those five pounds were from fat? Think about it. It could have been 2 pounds of muscle, 2 pounds of water, and 1 pound of fat. If this is the case, you are now in a worse situation than you were before the 5-pound loss. Why? Because your metabolism will end up being slower and you will have lost body shape (muscle is what increases your metabolism and also gives shape to your body). This is why crash diets don't work. They cause you to lose mostly muscle and water, while simultaneously creating fat storage. These diets trick the body into thinking that it is starving, so it begins storing fat for future use and eating away at valuable muscle. So while you may achieve your ideal *weight,* you'll look very different than what you envisioned.

Therefore, in order to achieve the look that you desire, forget about reaching your so-called ideal bodyweight. We humans are made up of simply too many varying frames and sizes, making it impossible to determine universal weight standards. Just follow the guidelines prescribed in Body Sculpting Diet (page 29) and let the fat calipers, tape measure, and the mirror tell you when you have arrived at your destination.

AVOID THE FADS

Every time we turn on the TV we are bombarded with the latest fad to lose fat and achieve the body of our dreams in only five minutes a day. All we need to do is buy some fancy new machine (that may be as "cheap" as three small credit card installments of $75.99), take some "magic" pills, or go on a "new" diet, and that dream body will be ours in record time. But we've all seen how far those promises got us.

If you've ever bought one of those "body in a box" gadgets or machines, recall the process that took place when you received it. You used it for a few weeks, if at all, right? Eventually it ends up becoming a great place to lay your clothes. The only thing that ends up losing weight in this case is your wallet.

With so many diets, gadgets, and magic potions available to us, it is no wonder that people become confused about how to properly get in shape. This is one of the major reasons why we decided to put together *The Body Sculpting Bible for Women Workout Journal.* We are sick and tired of seeing and hearing about how people are constantly being ripped off by these "get fit quick" schemes and hokey solutions that provide nothing more than another pile of junk. In addition, having dealt with weight problems ourselves, we naturally relate to people who want desperately to change the way they look but don't know how to go about doing so.

We will show you that you can lose fat very easily without starving yourself. In fact, you may end up eating more than you ever have in your life and still achieve the perfectly shaped physique you are looking for! We will also show you how to look great without having to exercise for hours a day. You don't even need to join a health club if you don't want to.

Our goal is to share with you all of the knowledge that we have accumulated in our combined 40 years of fitness experience in training both ourselves and women just like you. With this newfound knowledge you will soon be in total control of how you look and feel. No longer will it be a dreadful experience to step on the scale, try on those skinny jeans, or put on that little black dress that stopped fitting long ago. No longer will you be at the mercy of an infomercial because you'll know exactly what to do in order to look the way you want.

Now that we've laid out our goals, let's go and learn about how you can reach yours.

Everyone who has followed our program to the letter has achieved the body of their dreams. We have trained hundreds of thousands of people who have experienced success and now it is your turn! Everything is spelled out for you in *The Body Sculpting Bible for Women Workout Journal,* so there is no reason to fail! The power to succeed is within you!

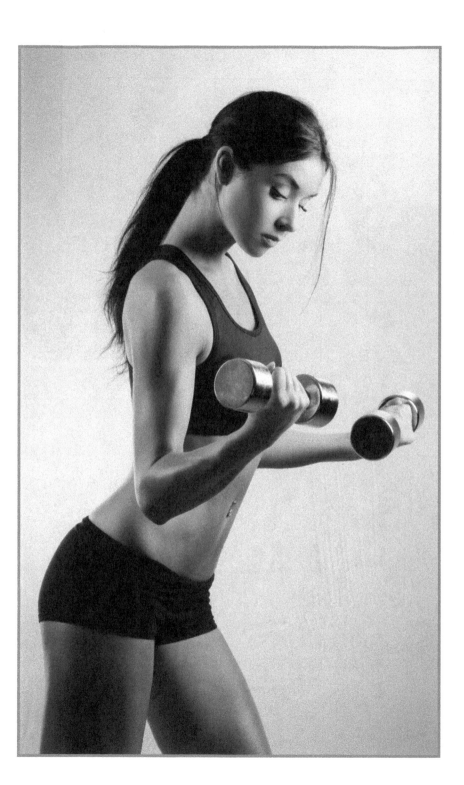

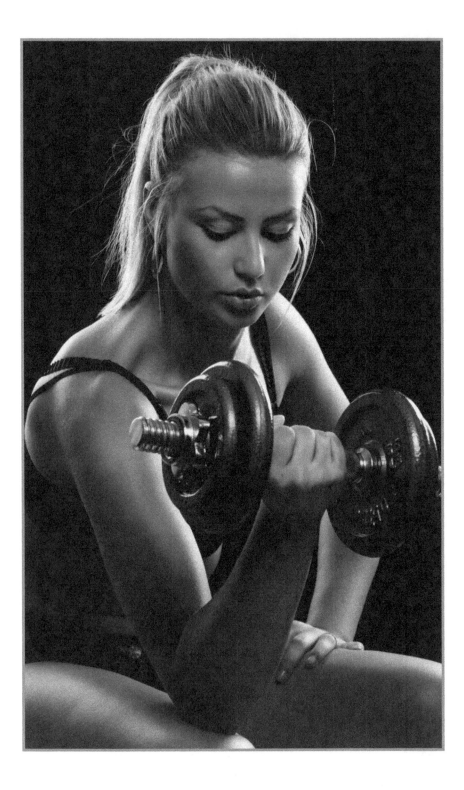

Guidelines to Body Sculpting Success

In this section, we give you some guidelines to help you reach your fitness goals. Follow these tips and you will be well on your way to achieving the body you've always dreamed of!

GUIDELINE #1: CREATE BODY SCULPTING GOALS

Without goals we are like a ship in the middle of the sea, just drifting away with no sense of direction. It just goes with the flow, so to speak, and if it ever gets anywhere it is just by mere accident. In order to achieve success from your body sculpting program, your goal should be clearly defined and engrained in your brain. Otherwise, like the drifting boat, if you get any-where it will be by mere chance. In this book, we will help you set goals and show you the map that will guide you from point A to point B.

GUIDELINE #2: FOLLOW A SENSIBLE BODY SCULPTING PROGRAM

Oftentimes, body sculpters who are just getting started will choose a rou-tine that is too advanced for their level, or simply go to the gym without any training plan. Taking on too much too soon can lead to injury and just going from machine to machine without any set routine will lead to mar-ginal results at best.

Others who are super motivated start to train 2-3 hours each day. However, anything over 1 hour leads to increased cortisol levels. Cortisol is a stress hormone that when secreted in excess will make you lose muscle and store body fat—not exactly the kind of results you are looking for. When it comes to fat loss and body sculpting, more is not necessarily bet-ter. You need to train hard, but also train smart.

Follow a sensible routine that fits your training level and the amount of time you can consistently dedicate to your endeavors and exe-cute it day in and day out. In this book you will find various routines rang-ing from beginner to advanced, as well as routines under 30 minutes for those of you who have very little time for exercise.

GUIDELINE #3: FOLLOW A SENSIBLE BODY SCULPTING DIET

Without the right diet to go along with your training program, you may find it difficult to lose body fat and gain muscle. Nutrition is what gives us the raw materials for recuperation, energy, and growth.

How many times we have seen people with the best intentions who are misled and fall for the latest fad diet. The end result most of the time is a rebound at the end of the program. Why is that? Because fad diets do not work *with* your body. They work *against* it by creating a drastic caloric deficit, which in turn, causes the body to lose muscle and react by lowering its metabolism. Furthermore, with the way these fad diets are created, even if they worked, there is no way you could stay on them forever.

Proper nutrition will work *with* your body by nourishing it and gently pushing it to lose fat as muscle tone is being built. In this manner, the end result will be a fit physique with a higher metabolic rate. This is the key to permanent results. The other thing to remember is that you need a program that you can live with since part of being able to achieve permanent results is to follow a program that you can stick to forever. In The Body Sculpting Diet (page 29), you will find a section on the Characteristics of a Good Nutrition Plan and with those principles (as well as the nutrition plans in that section), you will be able to get the permanent results you are looking for.

GUIDELINE #4: DON'T EXPECT BODYBUILDING SUPPLEMENTS TO DO ALL THE WORK FOR YOU

Supplements do not make up for improper training, or lack thereof, and/or a low-quality diet. Nutritional supplements only work when your diet and your training program are optimal. Keep in mind that supplements are just additions to an already good nutrition and training program. Once all of those aspects of your program are maximized, then you can start thinking of adding some supplements to your program.

Trust us when we say that we have tried everything out there and there are only a few supplements that you need to be concerned with. We will cover these later on in Body Sculpting Supplements (page 47). However, please listen to our advice: *do not* fall for the marketing hype that you see on TV, on the Internet, or in magazines of supplements that promise results in terms of fat loss and muscle gain with little or no work. If it were that easy, we would be the first ones taking such supplement and we would not be putting together this book, would we?

GUIDELINE #5: GET PROPER REST AND RECOVERY

Muscle gain and fat loss happen while you sleep. Surprised? The reason for that is because during sleep, your body releases all of the hormones that work to repair broken tissues. Therefore, sleep deprivation will cost you valuable body sculpting gains.

Ensure a good night's sleep every night and avoid staying up late if you don't need to in order to keep cortisol levels low.

Here are some tips on how to achieve a good night's sleep:

Avoid activities that involve deep concentration or high physical exertion. These activities will increase adrenaline levels and will prevent your body and brain from achieving the state of relaxation required to achieve sleep. Therefore, try to manage your time in such a way that your deep concentration activities as well as exercise are completed no later than 2 hours before going to bed.

Avoid watching disturbing shows at night on TV. This may also increase your adrenaline levels, thereby preventing you from enjoying a good night's sleep. In addition, these types of shows may also prompt your brain to start thinking and analyzing, thus preventing you from achieving a relaxed state.

Avoid eating a large meal at night. Since having a large meal requires time to digest, this will also prevent you from falling asleep. In addition, laying down in bed immediately after a big meal interferes with the digestion process, so not only will you not be able to fall asleep on time, but you won't be able to digest the food as you should either.

Attempt to totally relax at the same time each night. By doing so you condition the body to relax itself once the specific time that you choose comes every day. Ensure that at this time no thoughts other than relaxation and falling asleep come to your head. You need to really learn how to block all thoughts concerning work or other life issues that may be trying to get in your head. Listening to soothing music set at a low volume with the lights off can help you relax and achieve the state necessary to go to sleep.

HOW MUCH SLEEP DO YOU NEED?

While this greatly varies from person to person, ideally 7 to 8 hours of sleep each night on the average is what is needed. Some people need a bit more (up to 9) while others can do great with just 6. A simple rule of thumb is that if you find yourself consistently wanting to fall asleep during the day, then you need more sleep.

Sleeping well will not only keep you healthy and more energetic, but also will ensure that your body sculpting gains keep on coming.

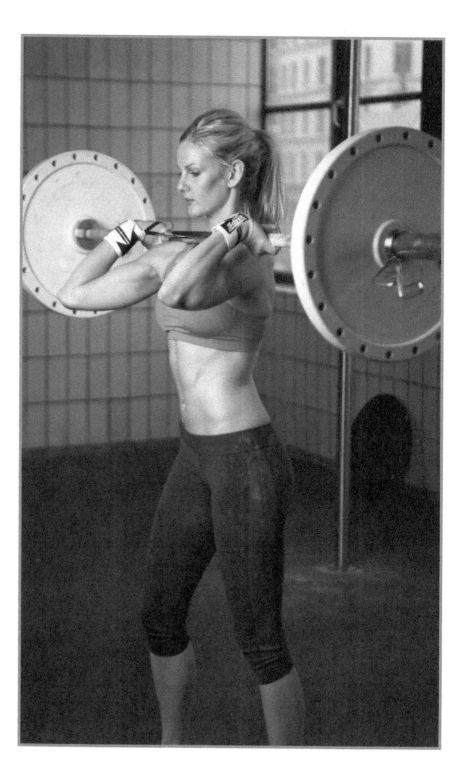

Setting Goals

In order to achieve success from the Body Sculpting Program, your goals should be clearly defined and engrained in your brain. Otherwise, your progress will be slow and you will find it difficult to stay motivated.

Have you ever noticed that some people go to the gym year after year but they still look the same and don't seem to be getting any results? I have approached people like that and asked them about their goals. In most cases, they don't have a clear definition of what they want. If you don't know where your target is, how can you hope to shoot at it and achieve it?

As a brief exercise, I would like you to think about and write down your long-term goals and your short-term goals.

YOUR LONG-TERM GOALS

Be specific! Write the measurements you want to have (chest, arms, thighs, calves, waist, hips), your body fat percentage, and your total body weight. Please, don't limit yourself to what you *think* you can achieve; write down what you *want* to achieve long-term.

My long-term body sculpting goal is to have measurements of:
Chest   _____
Arms   _____
Thighs   _____
Calves   _____
Waist   _____
Hips   _____
Body Fat %   _____
Weight   _____

Now, the problem is that such goals look so far away. Remember, every long trip starts with the first step, so now I want you to write your short-term goals.

YOUR SHORT-TERM GOALS

Short-term goals should be analyzed every 6 weeks. Obviously, short-term goals are going to be smaller than long term goals. However, by adding smaller short-term goals, you will get to your long-term goals in due time. When you write down your goals, be positive and have no doubt in your mind that you can achieve them. This is crucial!

For the next 6 weeks I will:

    Lose   _____ pounds of fat
    Gain   _____ pounds of muscle
    Weigh   _____ pounds

Have measurements of:

    Chest   _____
    Arms   _____
    Thighs   _____
    Calves   _____
    Waist   _____
    Hips   _____

ACTION PLAN

Once you have all of those goals written down, write down what action will you take for the next 6 weeks to get there. For instance:

- I will eat 4-6 balanced meals every day (1 every two to three hours).
- I will wake up to exercise and do cardio first thing in the morning three times each week.
- I will do 3-6 weight training sessions each week.
- I will get 8 hours of sleep (7 minimum) every day.
- I will drink a minimum of 1/2 gallon of water every day.

We also urge you to take pictures of how you currently look (be sure to also document your current measurements, bodyweight, body fat, etc.) and take progress pictures every two weeks. This is a great way to stay motivated because when you look at your beginner pictures, and then you look at pictures of yourself after six weeks, 12 weeks, six months, and a year later, you will see a huge difference!

Now that you have written all of this down, it is time to get to your actions. If you follow your action plan religiously and you miss your goals by a bit, *don't get discouraged!* You should have seen some progress anyway (here is where pictures really pay off; get a digital camera or use a smart phone) and this is what we are shooting for; constant progress is what will get you to the goals you want.

If you missed the mark due to the fact that you did not follow your action plan to the letter, don't punish yourself for it. Just set your new goals and be more determined in following your action plan so that you will get there this time.

If you mess up your plan for a day, don't drop the whole thing and quit! If you encounter one of those days, just recover the following day by starting the plan again.

Now that you have your goals in mind and have created your action plan, go ahead and put that plan into practice so that you can achieve your perfect body.

HERE IS A LIST OF WAYS THAT YOU CAN AVOID FITNESS FAILURE AND MAKE YOUR BODY SCULPTING GOALS A REALITY:

1. Create a scare tactic for yourself.

2. Find an accountability partner.

3. Make sure that your regimen includes the "Five Muscular Tiers," which are: Resistance Training, Cardiovascular Training, Nutrition, Supplementation, and Rest & Recuperation. By following the Body Sculpting Bible Program, you will fulfill this requirement.

4. Don't start your fitness regimen on New Years Day. It's a trend and trends end. Start it either before or after the holiday. Even a week apart is better than starting on this infamous day of destined fitness failures!

5. Be realistic with your goals. If you shoot too high, you could easily become frustrated and quit. Shoot for a doable goal, e.g. "I will lose three pounds by the end of this week" or "I will take my treadmill training to another level this week by increasing the speed by ½ MPH and adding a one-grade incline."

6. Make a pact with your family members. If you don't, self sabotage is imminent. If you all make fitness a part of your lives, all of your lives will surely be enriched.

THE 10 COMMANDMENTS OF BODY SCULPTING PERFECTION

Commandment #1: Believe in Yourself! If not, you won't be able to achieve your desired results!

Commandment #2: Write down your goals. How can you get somewhere if you don't know where you are heading?

Commandment #3: Set new goals every six weeks. After six weeks, compare your results against your original goals.

Commandment #4: Place a calendar on your fridge. Mark a back slash on the days that you followed your diet without cheating. Make a forward slash on the days that you trained. If you trained and followed a good diet on a given day, you should have an X marked on that day.

Commandment #5: Place a picture of how you currently look somewhere that you will be able to see on a daily basis. This picture should provide you with additional motivation to follow this program.

Commandment #6: Take pictures of yourself every 4 weeks and place them on the refrigerator next to your "before" picture. That way, whenever you have a craving and go to the refrigerator you will remember the reason that you are doing this and also get motivated by seeing what you're achieving.

Commandment #7: Write down the reasons why you are following this program and put them on your refrigerator. Same benefit as item 6.

Commandment #8: Keep your house free from any foods that are not good for your program. Only on Sundays can you bring these foods in the house.

Commandment #9: Remember to prepare all your meals the day before. If you bring your food with you to work, you are less likely to give in to your temptations.

Commandment #10: Remember that only you control what goes in your mouth. Food does not control you!

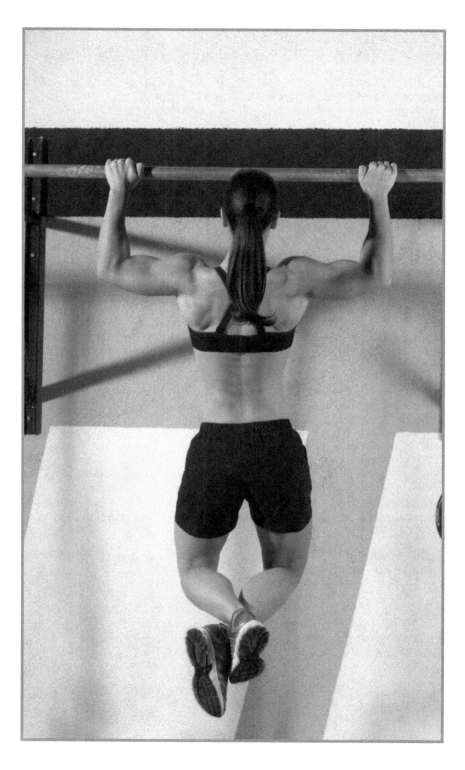

The Body Sculpting Training Program

Now that you have set your goals, it is time to come up with a plan to reach them. In order for you to be successful with your Body Sculpting Program, you need to first and foremost have the determination required to stick to the plan that will make you reach your goals. If you are not determined enough, then I am afraid that you will fail. Once you find that determination within you, then we need to look at the main components of the body sculpting equation which are training, nutrition, supplementation, and rest/recovery.

CHARACTERISTICS OF GOOD BODYBUILDING WEIGHT TRAINING ROUTINES

They must be short (between 45 to 60 minutes maximum). After about 60 minutes, the levels of muscle toning and fat burning hormones that your body produces (such as testosterone) begin to drop and cortisol levels (a stress hormone that preserves fat and eats up muscle) rise. What this means is that training more than 45 to 60 minutes will actually prevent you from gaining muscle tone and losing fat fast! It will also prevent you from fast recovery. As crazy as it sounds, that is the way it is.

The rest in between sets should be kept to a minimum (90 seconds or less). Limiting your rest in between sets and exercises not only helps you to perform a lot of work and still finish within the allotted time frame, but it also helps improve your cardiovascular system. In addition, it has been shown that this kind of training stimulates higher output of growth hormones.

Generally, the sets should be between 8 - 15 repetitions each (except for calves and abs). There are many reasons for this, including:
- Since you are doing so many repetitions, there is less probability of injury since you'll be using a weight that you can control.
- Studies show that muscle toning and fat burning occur more efficiently at these repetition ranges.

Training must be varied and cycled. Please, don't get stuck with the same routine day in and day out. If you do this, it will guarantee zero progress. This is without even mentioning boredom and lack of enthusiasm. If you don't know how to vary your program, there is no need to worry as all of the routines detailed in Body Sculpting Workouts (page 51) (and in all of the books in our *Body Sculpting Bible* series) detail exactly what you need to do on a daily basis.

Basic exercises should be the mainstay of your training program. Multi-jointed free weight exercises recruit many more muscle fibers than single-jointed exercises or machines. Therefore, these should compose the majority of your weight training routine.

In Body Sculpting Workouts (page 51), your workout routines (and we give you plenty to choose from) will be completely spelled out for you so there will be no guesswork on your part. Simply follow the workouts, log your progress in the Training Journal, and watch your body transform!

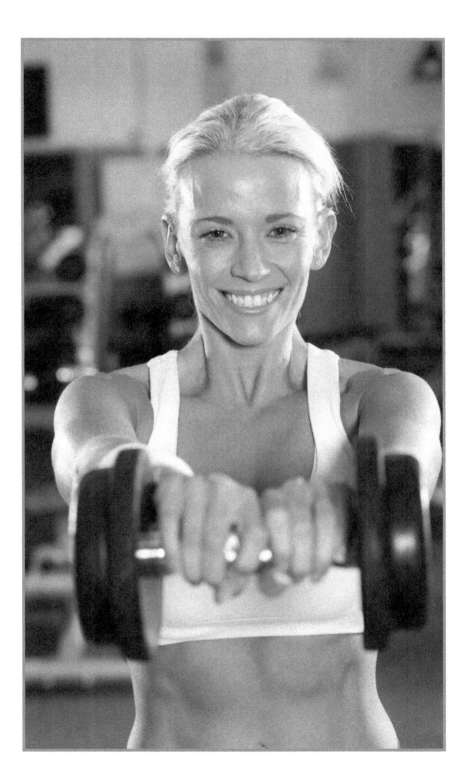

The Body Sculpting Diet

Training is what sparks the stimuli in the body that gives you the tone you are looking for. However, nutrition is what provides the raw materials for muscle toning and fat loss. As a matter of fact, the reason that many people go to the gym and still don't achieve results is because their nutrition is not what it should be.

CHARACTERISTICS OF A GOOD NUTRITION PROGRAM

It should favor smaller and frequent feedings throughout the day instead of large and infrequent ones. Why? Frequent feedings are of particular importance because after three to four hours without food, your body switches to a catabolic state; a state in which you lose muscle and gain fat. The body believes that it is starving and it starts feeding itself on lean muscle tissue and prepares to store calories as fat. Bad scenario! Losing muscle not only will prevent you from achieving the toned physique you are looking for, but it will also decrease your metabolism (making it easier for you to gain fat).

Therefore, in order for your program to work, you should eat four to six meals (depending on your goals) every day, spaced out at 2-1/2 to 3 hour intervals.

Every meal should have carbohydrates, protein, and fat in the correct ratios. Having a meal that is not balanced (for example, if your meal is all carbohydrates) won't yield the desired results. Every macronutrient has to be present in order for the body to absorb them and use them properly. Without boring you with the effect of food on the body's biochemistry, let's just say that if you only eat carbohydrates in one meal without anything else, your energy levels will crash in about 30 minutes and your body will be storing any carbohydrates that were not used into fat. Conversely, if you only eat protein, you will lack energy and your body will not be able to turn the protein into muscle because it is difficult for the body to absorb protein in the absence of carbohydrates. In addition, the ratios for each particular macronutrient must be correct in order to get the results you want. The ratio of your diet will look like the following:
- 40% carbohydrates
- 40% protein
- 20% fats

(Note that for every serving of carbohydrates, you get a serving of protein.)

The calories should be cycled. I strongly believe in caloric cycling as this will not allow the metabolism to get used to a certain caloric level, which leads to stagnant results.

Some weeks you will consume higher calories than others as you will see in the sample diets later in this section. These caloric intakes assume a normal activity level that only includes body sculpting training. Those of you involved in activities like marathon running or jobs requiring heavy physical labor will need to adjust your calories upwards accordingly (mainly in the form of carbohydrates) in order to support your higher levels of activity. In addition, those of you who are naturally skinny and are interested in only gaining muscle tone will need to have a higher carbohydrate intake.

NUTRITION BASICS

There are three macronutrients that the human body needs in order to function properly. These are carbohydrates, protein, and fats.

CARBOHYDRATES

Carbohydrates are your body's main source of energy. When you ingest carbohydrates, your pancreas releases a hormone called insulin. Insulin is very important because:
1) It grabs the carbohydrates and either stores them in the muscle or stores them as fat.
2) It grabs the amino acids (protein) and shelters them inside the muscle cell for recovery and repair.

While the above is an oversimplification of the many actions of insulin, for our purposes of discussion those are its main functions.

Most people who are overweight and are in low fat/high carbohydrate diets got into that condition because they are eating an overabundance of carbohydrates. Eating too many carbohydrates causes a huge release of insulin. When there is too much insulin in the body, your body turns into a fat storing machine because insulin is a great fat storing hormone. Therefore, in order to maximize your muscle gains, maintain stable energy levels, and have good fat loss, your insulin levels must remain steady and low.

It is important that you eat no more carbohydrates than necessary and that you eat the right amount of carbohydrates.

Now that we have talked about the importance of having just the right amount of carbohydrates, let's talk about which are the best sources of carbohydrates.

Complex Carbohydrates

You should be eating complex carbs in small portions (portion size depends on your body type), but more frequently throughout the day.

1) Starchy: Old-fashioned oatmeal, potatoes, plain pasta, rice (preferably brown rice), shredded wheat, yams, whole wheat bread, and corn.
2) Fibrous: Asparagus, squash, broccoli, green beans, cabbage, cauliflower, celery, cucumber, mushrooms, lettuce, red or green peppers, tomato, spinach, and zucchini.

Simple Carbohydrates

You should be eating simple carbs sparingly, primarily in the morning and after your exercise session. Good sources of simple carbs include: Bananas, grapes, yogurt, apples, cantaloupe, strawberries, and skim milk (also contains protein).

PROTEIN

Every tissue in your body is made up of protein (including muscle, hair, skin, and nails). Proteins are the building blocks of lean muscle tissue. Without it, building muscle and burning fat efficiently would be impossible. Because of this, its importance is paramount. Protein helps increase your metabolism by 20-30 percent every time you eat it, and it time-releases carbohydrates (glucose) to give you sustained energy throughout the day.

You should consume between 1-1.5 grams of protein per pound of lean body mass. In other words, if you weigh 130 pounds and have 16% body fat, you should consume at least 109 grams of protein, since your lean body mass is 109 pounds. Nobody should consume more than 1.5 grams per pound of lean body mass as this is unnecessary and the extra protein will either be converted to glucose, excreted out of the body, or worse, provide excess calories that may get stored as fat.

Good sources of protein include: White Fish, halibut, cod, lean round steak, chicken breast, tuna (in spring water), turkey breast, whey protein, and skim milk (also contains simple carbs).

FATS

All the cells in the body have some fat in them. Fats are responsible for lubricating your joints. In addition, hormones are manufactured from fats. If you eliminate all fats from your diet, your hormonal production will drop and a whole array of chemical reactions will be interrupted. Your body will start accumulating more body fat than usual to keep functioning. Because your testosterone production is halted, the production of lean muscle mass will be interrupted as well. Therefore, in order to have an efficient metabolism, you need to consume certain fats. There are three types of fats: Saturated, polyunsaturated, and monounsaturated.

Saturated Fats

Saturated fats are associated with heart disease and high cholesterol levels. However, you do need a small amount of natural saturated fats in your diet to support health and hormonal production. The best way to obtain your daily requirement of saturated fat is from egg yolks. Just 1-2 whole eggs every day will add the saturated fat that the body needs in order to function properly. On the other hand, the fats that have absolutely no place in your diet are trans fats or partially hydrogenated oils. What are partially hydrogenated oils? These are saturated fats that have been altered chemically through the addition of extra hydrogen atoms. This chemical manipulation gives these fats unnatural properties that foster fat gain, insulin insensitivity (the cells in your body lose the ability to let insulin inside them so that the much needed nutrients like amino acids, glucose and other fats can nourish the cell), blocked arteries, and a whole myriad of other issues. In addition, it is much harder to burn off these fats because they have a melting temperature that is much higher than that of normal fats. Just to put it in perspective, oleic acid has a melting point of 13.4°C (56°F) while a trans fat has a melting point of 45°C (113°F). While that is great for dramatically extending the shelf life of food items, how can our bodies (which normally operate at around 37°C) be expected to burn these fats? Food for thought. I wholeheartedly believe that trans fats are one of the reasons why we see so much heart disease, high cholesterol, diabetes and even cancer these days. Consider these as poison and always stay away from processed foods.

Polyunsaturated Fats

Polyunsaturated fats are fats that do not have an effect on cholesterol levels. Most of the fats in vegetable oils (such as corn, cottonseed, safflower, soybean, and sunflower oil) are polyunsaturated. However, the best polyunsaturated fats are fish oils and flaxseed oil, which are extremely high in essential fatty acids and have incredible anti-inflammatory properties as well as many other benefits such as increased fat burning!

Monounsaturated Fats

Monounsaturated fats have a positive effect on the good cholesterol levels. The best sources of monounsaturated fats are: extra virgin olive oil and nuts like cashews, almonds, and peanuts.

Twenty percent of your calories should come from good fats. If good fats make up any less than 20% of your diet, your hormonal production will go down. If more than 20% of your diet is made up of fats, you will start accumulating more fat on your body. The best sources of fat to consume are extra virgin olive oil, nuts, fish oils, flaxseed oil, and some saturated fats from egg yolks (1-2 per day).

WATER

Water is by far the most abundant substance in our bodies. Without water, an organism would not survive very long. Most people who come to me for advice on how to get in shape almost always underestimate the value of water. Water is good for the following reasons:

- Over 65% of your body is composed of water (most of the muscle cell is water).
- Water cleanses your body from toxins and pollutants that would make you sick.
- Water is needed for all of the complex chemical reactions that your body needs to perform on a daily basis. Processes such as energy production, muscle building, and fat burning require water. A lack of water would interrupt all of these processes.
- Water helps lubricate the joints.
- When the outside temperature rises, water serves as a coolant to bring the body temperature down to where it is supposed to be.
- Water helps control your appetite. Sometimes when you feel hungry after a good meal this sensation indicates a lack of water. Drinking water at that time will help take the craving away.
- Cold water increases your metabolism.

In order to know how much water your body needs in a day, just multiply your lean body mass by .66. For example, if you weigh 130 pounds and have 16% body fat, your lean body mass is 109 pounds. 109 x .66 = 71.94, so you would need to drink approximately 72 ounces of water each day.

THE 14-DAY BODY SCULPTING DIET PLAN

Presented below is the 14-Day Body Sculpting Diet Plan. For the first two weeks, you will follow the Low Calorie Diet and for the next two weeks, you will follow the High Calorie Diet. For best results, stick to the choices presented in the Approved Lists.

WEEKS 1-2: CALORIES:LOW (Approximately 1200 calories)

Around 120 grams of carbohydrates (mostly complex with simple carbs being saved for after the workout)

Around 120 grams of protein

Around 26 grams of fats

MEAL #1 (7:30 AM) BREAKFAST (POST-WORKOUT)
Choose 1 serving of Proteins
Choose 1 serving of Starchy Carbs
Optionally, you may choose to add 1 serving of Simple Carbs in the form of Fruit, if you can't live without them.

MEAL #2 (10:30 AM) MORNING BREAK SNACK
Choose 1 serving of Proteins
Choose 1 serving of Starchy Carbs
Choose 1 serving of Good Fats

MEAL #3 (1:30 PM) LUNCH TIME
Choose 1 serving of Proteins
Choose 1 serving of Starchy Carbs
Choose 1 serving of Fibrous Carbs
Choose 1 serving of Good Fats

MEAL #4 (3:30 PM) AFTERNOON BREAK SNACK
Choose 1 serving of Proteins
Choose 1 serving of Starchy Carbs

MEAL #5 (6:30 PM) DINNER
Choose 1 serving of Proteins
Choose 1/2 serving of Starchy Carbs
Choose 1 serving of Fibrous Carbs
Choose 1 serving of Good Fats

WEEKS 3-4 CALORIES: HIGH (Approximately 1500 calories)

150 grams of carbohydrates (mostly complex with simple carbs being saved for after the workout)

150 grams of protein

33 grams of fats

MEAL #1 (7:30 AM) BREAKFAST (POST-WORKOUT)
Choose 1 serving of Proteins
Choose 1 serving of Starchy Carbs
Optionally, you may choose to add 1 serving of Simple Carbs in the form of Fruit, if you can't live without them.

MEAL #2 (10:30 AM) MORNING BREAK SNACK
Choose 1 serving of Proteins
Choose 1 serving of Starchy Carbs

MEAL #3 (1:30 PM) LUNCH TIME
Choose 1 serving of Proteins
Choose 1 serving of Starchy Carbs
Choose 1 serving of Fibrous Carbs
Choose 1 serving of Good Fats

MEAL #4 (3:30 PM) AFTERNOON BREAK SNACK
Choose 1 serving of Proteins
Choose 1 serving of Starchy Carbs

MEAL #5 (6:30 PM) DINNER
Choose 1 serving of Proteins
Choose 1/2 serving of Starchy Carbs
Choose 1 serving of Fibrous Carbs
Choose 1 serving of Good Fats

MEAL #6 (8:30 PM) LATE SNACK
Choose 1 serving of Proteins
Choose 1/2 serving of Starchy Carbs
Choose 1 serving of Fibrous Carbs
Choose 1 serving of Good Fats

Nutrition Chart and Glycemic Index

STARCHY CARBOHYDRATES			
Eat with all 5-6 meals throughout the day. Around 25-27 grams of carbohydrates per serving. 1 serving per meal.			
FOOD ITEM	SERVING SIZE (MEASURE DRY)	GLYCEMIC INDEX	DESIRABLE
Old Fashioned Oats	1/2 cup dry	Low	Highly
Cream of Rice	1/4 cup dry	High	Good After Workout Only
Cream of Wheat	4 tablespoons dry	Medium	Good
Baked Potatoes	4 ounces cooked	Medium	Good
Sweet Potatoes	4 ounces cooked	Medium	Good
Rice (Brown Whole Grain)	1/2 cup cooked	Medium	Good
White Rice	1/2 cup cooked	High	Good After Workout Only
Spaghetti	4 oz cooked	Low	Good in GI but too many carbs for a small serving.
Whole wheat flour bread	2 slices	High	Not a great choice but okay in moderation.
Corn	3/4 cup	Medium	Good
Peas	1 cup	Medium	Good
Low GI=1-55 Medium GI=56-69 High GI=70-100			

SIMPLE CARBOHYDRATES			
If you must, eat 1 serving with Breakfast and 1 after workout as even though they are low to medium in GI, too many simple sugars from fruits in the diet throughout the day can prevent fat loss. If your post workout meal is breakfast, then just consume 1 serving per day of fruits. Around 10 grams of carbohydrates per serving. If breakfast is the post workout meal: 1 serving per day with post workout meal. If post workout meal is not breakfast: 1 serving with breakfast and 1 serving with post workout meal.			
FOOD ITEM	SERVING SIZE	GLYCEMIC INDEX	DESIRABLE
Apples	1/2	Low	Good
Oranges	1/2	Low	Good
Grapefruit	1/2	Low	Good
Cherries	7	Low	Good
Pears	1/3	Low	Good
Bananas	1/3	Medium	After Workout Only
Lemons	1	Low	Good
Cantaloupe	1/4 melon	High	After Workout Only
Strawberries	1 cup	1 cup	Good
Apricots	3	Medium	After Workout Only
Grapes	1/2 cup	Low	Good
Mango	1/3 cup	Medium	After Workout Only
Papaya	1/2 cup	Medium	After Workout Only
Low GI=1-55 Medium GI=56-69 High GI=70-100			

FIBROUS CARBOHYDRATES

Eat at least 1 serving with lunch and 1 serving with dinner though more can be consumed if desired; consider these free foods as they do not get absorbed.

Around 10 grams of carbohydrates per serving. At least 1 serving at lunch and 1 serving at dinner.

FOOD ITEM	SERVING SIZE (MEASURE COOKED)	GLYCEMIC INDEX	DESIRABLE
Broccoli	1 cup	Low	Good
Green Beans	1 cup	Low	Good
Asparagus	12 spears or 1 cup	Low	Good
Lettuce	1 head raw	Low	Good
Tomatoes	2 cups chopped	Low	Good
Green Peppers (chopped)	1-1/2 cups raw	Low	Good
Onions	1/2 cup	Low	Good
Mushrooms	1 cup	Low	Good
Cucumber sliced	3 cups	Low	Good
Cauliflower	2 cups	Low	Good
Spinach	4 cups	Low	Good
Cabbage	2 cups	Low	Good
Carrots	1/2 cup sliced	High	After Workout

Low GI=1-55 Medium GI=56-69 High GI=70-100

PROTEINS

Eat with all 5-6 meals throughout the day. Around 20-23 grams of protein per serving. 1 serving per meal.

FOOD ITEM	SERVING SIZE (MEASURE COOKED)	GLYCEMIC INDEX	DESIRABLE
Chicken breast (skinless)	3 ounces	Low	Good
Turkey	3 ounces	Low	Good
Veal	3 ounces	Low	Good
Top Sirloin	3 ounces	Low	Good
Tuna	3 ounces	Low	Good
Wild Alaskan Salmon	3 ounces	Low	Good
Egg Whites (in carton)	1 cup	Low	Good
Whey Protein	1 scoop	Low	Good
Orange Roughy	3 ounces	Low	Good

GOOD FATS

Around 5 grams of fats per serving. 1 serving at lunch, dinner, and any other meal except post workout meal.

FOOD ITEM	SERVING SIZE	GLYCEMIC INDEX	DESIRABLE
Fish Oils	1 teaspoon	Low	Good
Flax Oils	1 teaspoon	Low	Good
Extra Virgin Olive Oil	1 teaspoon	Low	Good
Natural Peanut Butter	2 teaspoons	Low	Good

All fats are low in glycemic index and by combining a carbohydrate with a protein the combined glycemic index of the whole meal goes down. The fats included here were selected due to their high essential fatty acids content and their health properties.

NOTES: Avoid cooking with flax oil as the heat degrades the oil. Bake and broil instead of frying. Also, if eating salmon, eliminate 2 servings of good fats as salmon is high on EFAs.

The complete list of the glycemic index and glycemic load for 750 foods can be found in the article "International tables of glycemic index and glycemic load values: 2002." by Kaye Foster-Powell, Susanna H.A. Holt, and Janette C. Brand-Miller in the July 2002 American Journal of Clinical Nutrition, Vol. 62, pages 5–56. <http://www.ajcn.org/cgi/content/full/76/1/5>

SAMPLE DIETS

These diets are samples of what you can eat on a daily basis. Remember that you don't have to be stuck to just what is written here. You can vary your daily plan by following the 14-Day Body Sculpting Diet Plan and using these daily menus as examples.

SAMPLE 14-DAY LOW-CALORIE MILK-FREE DIET
(THIS DIET IS GOOD FOR THOSE WHO WANT TO ELIMINATE MILK PRODUCTS FROM THEIR PROGRAM.)

MEAL #	FOOD	SERVING SIZE
MEAL 1 BREAKFAST (POST-WORKOUT) 7:30 AM	WHEY PROTEIN BANANA CREAM OF RICE	1 SCOOP 1/3 BANANA 1/4 CUP DRY
MEAL 2 10:30 AM	WHEY PROTEIN OLD-FASHIONED OATS FLAXSEED OIL	1 SCOOP 1/2 CUP (MEASURED DRY) 1 TEASPOON
MEAL 3 1:30 PM	BROWN RICE GREEN BEANS CHICKEN BREAST EXTRA-VIRGIN OLIVE OIL	1/2 CUP COOKED 1 CUP 3 OUNCES 1 TEASPOON
MEAL 4 3:30 PM	WHEY PROTEIN OLD-FASHIONED OATS	1 SCOOP 1/2 CUP (MEASURED DRY)
MEAL 5 6:30 PM	WILD ALASKAN SALMON SWEET POTATOES BROCCOLI	3 OUNCES 2 OUNCES COOKED 1 CUP

SAMPLE 14-DAY HIGH-CALORIE MILK-FREE DIET

(THIS DIET IS GOOD FOR THOSE WHO WANT TO ELIMINATE MILK PRODUCTS FROM THEIR PROGRAM.)

MEAL #	FOOD	SERVING SIZE
MEAL 1 BREAKFAST (POST-WORKOUT) 7:30 AM	WHEY PROTEIN BANANA CREAM OF RICE	1 SCOOP 1/3 BANANA 1/4 CUP DRY
MEAL 2 10:30 AM	WHEY PROTEIN OLD-FASHIONED OATS FLAXSEED OIL	1 SCOOP 1/2 CUP (MEASURED DRY) 1 TEASPOON
MEAL 3 1:30 PM	BROWN RICE GREEN BEANS CHICKEN BREAST EXTRA-VIRGIN OLIVE OIL	1/2 CUP COOKED 1 CUP 3 OUNCES 1 TEASPOON
MEAL 4 3:30 PM	WHEY PROTEIN OLD-FASHIONED OATS	1 SCOOP 1/2 CUP (MEASURED DRY)
MEAL 5 6:30 PM	WILD ALASKAN SALMON SWEET POTATOES BROCCOLI	3 OUNCES 2 OUNCES COOKED 1 CUP
MEAL 6 8:30 PM	ORANGE ROUGHY BAKED POTATOES ASPARAGUS FLAXSEED OIL	3 OUNCES 2 OUNCES 1 CUP 1 TEASPOON

SAMPLE 14-DAY LOW-CALORIE DIET WITH MILK PRODUCTS

MEAL #	FOOD	SERVING SIZE
MEAL 1 BREAKFAST (POST-WORKOUT) 7:30 AM	WHEY PROTEIN SKIM MILK CREAM OF RICE	1/2 SCOOP 8 OUNCES 1/4 CUP DRY
MEAL 2 10:30 AM	WHEY PROTEIN OLD-FASHIONED OATS SKIM MILK FLAXSEED OIL	1/2 SCOOP 1/4 CUP (MEASURED DRY) 8 OUNCES 1 TEASPOON
MEAL 3 1:30 PM	BROWN RICE GREEN BEANS CHICKEN BREAST EXTRA-VIRGIN OLIVE OIL	1/2 CUP COOKED 1 CUP 3 OUNCES 1 TEASPOON
MEAL 4 3:30 PM	WHEY PROTEIN OLD-FASHIONED OATS	1 SCOOP 1/2 CUP (MEASURED DRY)
MEAL 5 6:30PM	WILD ALASKAN SALMON SWEET POTATOES BROCCOLI	3 OUNCES 2 OUNCES COOKED 1 CUP

SAMPLE 14-DAY HIGH-CALORIE DIET WITH MILK PRODUCTS

MEAL #	FOOD	SERVING SIZE
MEAL 1 BREAKFAST (POST-WORKOUT) 7:30 AM	WHEY PROTEIN SKIM MILK CREAM OF RICE	1/2 SCOOP 8 OUNCES 1/4 CUP DRY
MEAL 2 10:30 AM	WHEY PROTEIN OLD-FASHIONED OATS SKIM MILK FLAXSEED OIL	1/2 SCOOP 1/4 CUP (MEASURED DRY) 8 OUNCES 1 TEASPOON
MEAL 3 1:30 PM	BROWN RICE GREEN BEANS CHICKEN BREAST EXTRA-VIRGIN OLIVE OIL	1/2 CUP COOKED 1 CUP 3 OUNCES 1 TEASPOON
MEAL 4 3:30 PM	WHEY PROTEIN OLD-FASHIONED OATS	1 SCOOP 1/2 CUP (MEASURED DRY)
MEAL 5 6:30 PM	WILD ALASKAN SALMON SWEET POTATOES BROCCOLI	3 OUNCES 2 OUNCES COOKED 1 CUP
MEAL 6 8:30 PM	ORANGE ROUGHY BAKED POTATOES ASPARAGUS FLAXSEED OIL	3 OUNCES 2 OUNCES COOKED 1 CUP 1 TEASPOON

SAMPLE 14-DAY LOW-CALORIE OVO-LACTO VEGETARIAN DIET

MEAL #	FOOD	SERVING SIZE
MEAL 1 BREAKFAST (POST-WORKOUT) 7:30 AM	WHEY PROTEIN SKIM MILK CREAM OF RICE	1/2 SCOOP 8 OUNCES 1/4 CUP DRY
MEAL 2 10:30 AM	WHEY PROTEIN OLD-FASHIONED OATS SKIM MILK FLAXSEED OIL	1/2 SCOOP 1/4 CUP (MEASURED DRY) 8 OUNCES 1 TEASPOON
MEAL 3 1:30 PM	BROWN RICE GREEN BEANS EGG WHITES EXTRA-VIRGIN OLIVE OIL	1/2 CUP COOKED 1 CUP 1 CUP 1 TEASPOON
MEAL 4 3:30 PM	WHEY PROTEIN OLD-FASHIONED OATS	1 SCOOP 1/2 CUP (MEASURED DRY)
MEAL 5 6:30 PM	EGG WHITES SWEET POTATOES BROCCOLI	1 CUP 2 OUNCES COOKED 1 CUP

SAMPLE 14-DAY HIGH-CALORIE OVO-LACTO VEGETARIAN DIET

MEAL #	FOOD	SERVING SIZE
MEAL 1 BREAKFAST (POST-WORKOUT) 7:30 AM	WHEY PROTEIN SKIM MILK CREAM OF RICE	1/2 SCOOP 8 OUNCES 1/4 CUP DRY
MEAL 2 10:30 AM	WHEY PROTEIN OLD-FASHIONED OATS SKIM MILK FLAXSEED OIL	1/2 SCOOP 1/4 CUP (MEASURED DRY) 8 OUNCES 1 TEASPOON
MEAL 3 1:30 PM	BROWN RICE GREEN BEANS EGG WHITES EXTRA-VIRGIN OLIVE OIL	1/2 CUP COOKED 1 CUP 1 CUP 1 TEASPOON
MEAL 4 3:30 PM	WHEY PROTEIN OLD-FASHIONED OATS	1 SCOOP 1/2 CUP (MEASURED DRY)
MEAL 5 6:30PM	EGG WHITES SWEET POTATOES BROCCOLI	1 CUP 2 OUNCES COOKED 1 CUP
MEAL 6 8:30 PM	EGG WHITES BAKED POTATOES ASPARAGUS FLAXSEED OIL	1 CUP 2 OUNCES COOKED 1 CUP 1 TEASPOON

GROCERY SHOPPING LIST

Always make sure to eat a meal prior to going grocery shopping to ensure that you don't buy junk foods. Another strategy is to do your grocery shopping on Sundays, when you are allowed to eat whatever you want for one meal. Obviously, you do not need to purchase all of the items on this grocery list. We provide it as a reminder of the types of foods that your shopping list should include.

CARBOHYDRATES

Brown rice

Chickpeas

Cream of rice

Yams (sweet potatoes)

Whole wheat bread

Plain oatmeal (old fashion, not instant)

Corn

Baking potato

Pita bread

Lentils

Grits

Fruits

Fresh green vegetables

PROTEINS

Chicken breasts (avoid deli meats; they are high in sodium and low in protein)

Turkey breasts (avoid deli meats; they are high in sodium and low in protein)

Water-packed Tuna

White fish

Eggs

Halibut

Cod

Round steak

Top sirloin

FATS

Flaxseed Oil

SUPPLEMENTS

Vitamin and mineral formula

Vitamin C

Chromium picolinate

Fish oil capsules (if you don't use flaxseed oil)

Meal replacement powders

Whey protein powders

Protein bars

Creatine

Glutamine

DAIRY

Skim Milk

MISCELLANEOUS ITEMS

Garlic powder (for flavoring)

Onion powder (for flavoring)

Balsamic vinegar

Crystal light

Any sugar-free and salt-free seasoning

(Photocopy these pages for your own personal use)

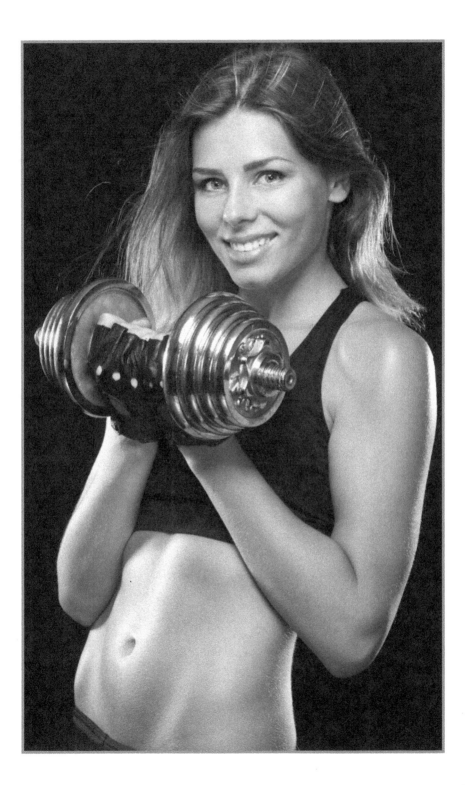

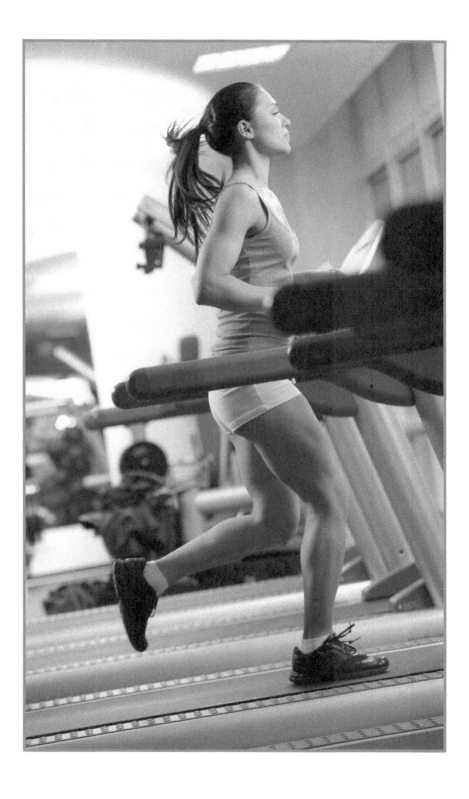

Body Sculpting Supplements

When it comes to losing fat and gaining lean muscle tone, many people think that supplements are the most important part of the equation. However, this could not be any further from the truth.

Supplements are just additions to a balanced nutrition and training program. Nutrition and training are the most important components of a body sculpting program, along with rest and recovery. Once all of those aspects of your program have been maximized, you can start adding supplements to your program.

Remember, supplements do not make up for improper training (or lack thereof) or a low quality diet. Supplements only work when your diet and your training program are optimal.

WHY USE SUPPLEMENTS?

Nutritional supplements are beneficial because they prevent nutritional deficiencies. The increased activity levels from your new exercise program will cause your body to need greater amounts of vitamins and minerals, which can increase the probability of you experiencing nutrient deficiencies without supplementation. Even a slight deficiency can sabotage fat loss and toning. Why can't we just get all the nutrients we need from the food we eat? We cannot rely solely on food to provide us with all the vitamins and minerals that our body needs because the processing of foods before they get to the supermarket, after cooking, and with exposure to air and light have already robbed your foods of many of the vitamins they would offer. If you are deficient in one or more nutrients your body may not be able to build muscle and burn fat properly.

However, not all supplements are created equal. There are some nutrients which your body always needs, while others are more dependent upon what your goals are and what your budget looks like. Below is a brief list of the supplements that are useful when training. For a full description of all these supplements, please refer to our book, *Body Sculpting Bible for Women.*

ESSENTIALS TO TAKE

- Multi-vitamin/mineral complex taken twice daily with breakfast.
- Protein shake taken after your workout (or with lunch on non-workout days).
- 3 capsules of fish oils taken with breakfast, lunch, and dinner (or 3-

6 teaspoons of flaxseed oil or Carlson fish oils if capsules are not desired).

- 1 gram of vitamin C taken with breakfast, lunch, and dinner.
- Protein powder (preferably a blend of various proteins) or meal replacement powder for mixing with skim milk or water in order to make protein shakes.
- 200 mcg of Chromium Picolinate taken with a protein shake after your workout.

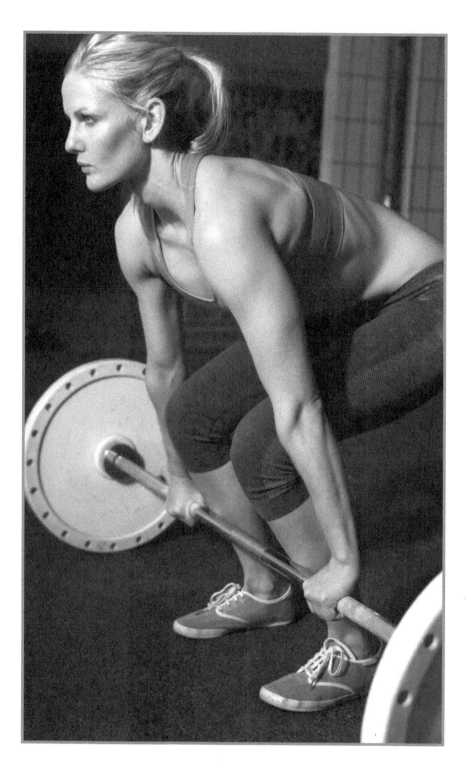

Body Sculpting Workouts

Choose from one of the many Body Sculpting Workouts in this section, based on your goals and experience level. If you have never trained before, start with the beginner Break-In Routine. Before each workout, be sure to start with the Stretching routine below.

Note: Please refer to the books in our *Body Sculpting Bible* series for the most complete exercise descriptions of how to perform the weight training exercises.

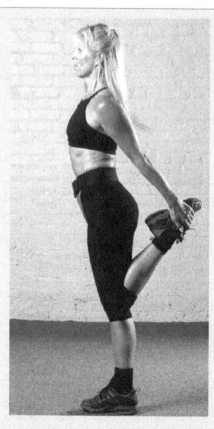
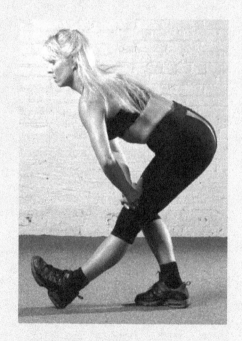

STRETCHING

Stretch your thighs by grasping a pole with one arm and bending the opposite leg, bringing your foot towards your buttocks (if you grasp the pole with the left hand, then bend the right leg). Grasp your ankle with the free hand and slowly lift your foot as comfortably as possible. Hold this position for a count of five and repeat with the oter leg.

Stretch your hamstrings by stepping forward with your left heel while bending your right knee. Keep your left leg straight and toe pointed up. Placing your hands on your left thigh, bend forward at the waist and feel the stretch in your hamstring. Hold this position for a count of five and repeat with the opposite leg.

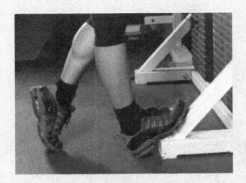

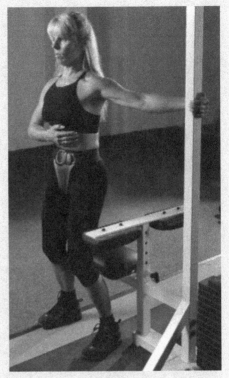

Stretch your calves by grasping a pole with both arms, standing on a raised surface, and placing one foot on the edge of the surface in order to allow your heel to go down as far as comfortably possible. Hold this position for a count of five and repeat with the other leg.

Stretch your chest by grasping a pole with one of your arms, ensuring that this arm is parallel to the ground. Slowly turn away from the pole and allow your arm to be as far behind the body as possible. Ensure that you do not overextend your chest by going as far away as is comfortably possible. Hold this position for a count of five and repeat with the other arm.

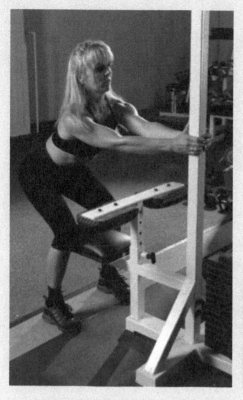

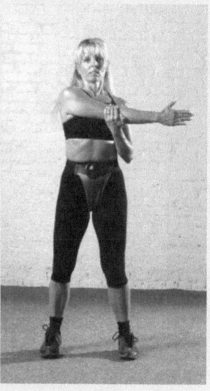

Stretch your back by grasping a pole with both arms, bending your knees, and sitting back in order to fully extend your arms and achieve a stretch in your lats and lower back. Hold this position for a count of five.

Stretch your shoulders by grasping one of your wrists with the opposite hand. Without moving your torso, begin to pull your arm as far as possible. Hold this position for a count of five and repeat with the other arm.

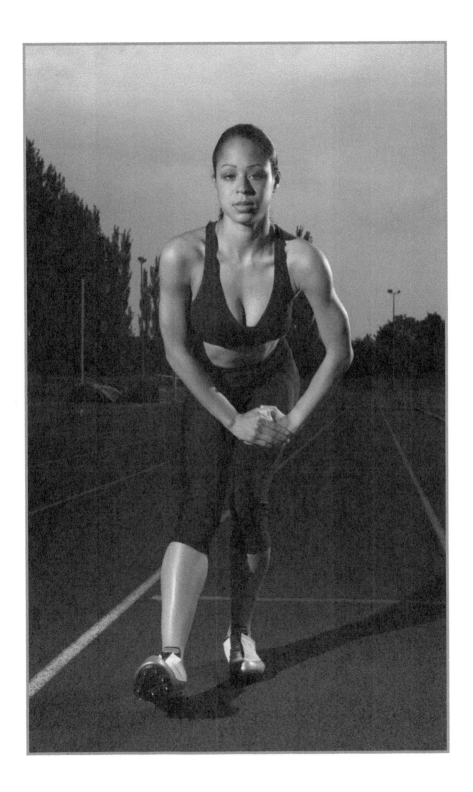

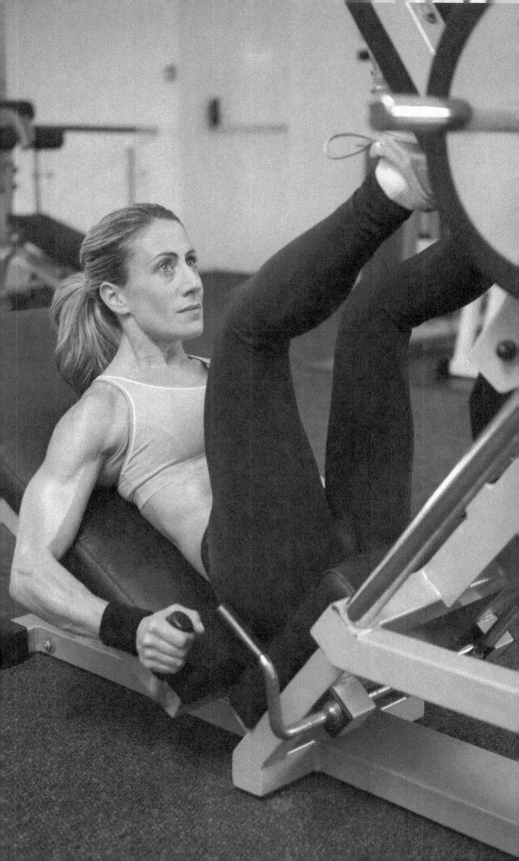

Break-In Routine

BREAK-IN ROUTINE

In this program you will train with weights three days a week and perform aerobic activity three days a week. In this book, we use Sunday as your day off. You may do Day 1 on Mondays, Day 2 on Wednesdays, Day 3 on Fridays, and Cardio with Abs on Tuesdays, Thursdays and Saturdays. Any other combination like Day 1 on Tuesdays, Day 2 on Thursdays, Day 3 on Saturdays, and Cardio with Abs on Wednesdays, Fridays and Sundays is also valid.

This program is designed to be performed in the comfort of your home with minimum equipment, namely a pair of dumbbells or a pair of dumbbells with an adjustable bench. As you get stronger you may wish to purchase a pair of secure adjustable dumbbells such as Powerblocks.

HOW TO PROGRESS WITH THE BREAK-IN ROUTINE

For the first six weeks, follow the routine exactly as it is laid out. If you have never worked out before, it will take your body approximately six weeks to get used to the movements and recruit muscle fibers. It will also give your cardiovascular system a chance to get used to this type of training. By the end of the six weeks, you should have lost a significant amount of weight and begin seeing more muscle tone and definition in your body. You should also be able to reach your target heart rate by the end of this period.

After week 6, add one more set to all of the exercises. You will now be performing three sets instead of two. Increase the weights and perform fewer repetitions (13-15, except for Abs and Calves where the repetition range stays the same). Also, increase your aerobic activity to 20 minutes. Follow this workout for the next 4 weeks.

After week 10, you are ready to go up to 4 sets per exercise and 30 minutes of cardio. Increase the weights and perform fewer repetitions (10-12, except for Abs and Calves where the repetition range stays the same). Also, reduce the rest between sets to 60 seconds. Follow this workout for three more weeks; you should not only look dramatically different, but now you will also be in shape to start the 14-Day Body Sculpting Program.

Break-In Routine

SPECIAL INSTRUCTIONS FOR WEEKS 1 & 2

Use modified compound supersets. Perform modified compound supersets by performing the first exercise, resting for the prescribed rest period, performing the second exercise, resting the prescribed rest period and going back to the first exercise. Continue in this manner until you have performed all of the prescribed number of sets, and then continue with the next modified compound superset. You will repeat Day 1 on Monday, Day 2 on Wednesday, and Day 3 on Friday.

DAY 1   MONDAY

EXERCISE	REPS	SETS	REST (seconds)
Dumbbell One-Arm Row	15-20	2	90
Push-Up (against wall if unable to perform on floor)	15-20	2	90
Dumbbell Shoulder Press	15-20	2	90
Standing Calf Raise (two legs)	15-20	2	90
Dumbbell Curl	15-20	2	90
Overhead Dumbbell Extension	15-20	2	90
Dumbbell Squat	15-20	2	90
Stiff-Legged Deadlift	15-20	2	90

NOTES ON PUSH-UPS

Depending on your body weight, you may find this exercise difficult to do in the traditional way. If this is the case, then start by performing them standing against the wall (stand 1.5-2 ft. in front of the wall, extend your arms and perform the exercise). In this position you will not be lifting your full bodyweight. As you become stronger, you may perform push-ups against the floor "from your knees." Once you master that position, you will be able to perform the traditional push-up.

DAY 2   WEDNESDAY

EXERCISE	REPS	SETS	REST (seconds)
Dumbbell Squat	15-20	2	90
Dumbbell Lunge	15-20	2	90
Ballet Squat	15-20	2	90
Stiff-Legged Deadlift	15-20	2	90
Standing Calf Raise (one leg)	15-20	2	90
Upright Row	15-20	2	90
Standing Calf Raise (two legs)	15-20	2	90
Triceps Kickback	15-20	2	90

DAY 3			FRIDAY
EXERCISE	REPS	SETS	REST (seconds)
MODIFIED COMPOUND SUPERSET # 1 — back — Two-Arm Row	15-20	2	90
chest — Flat Dumbbell Fly (lying on the floor) (against wall if unable to perform on floor)	15-20	2	90
MODIFIED COMPOUND SUPERSET # 2 — shoulders — Bent-Over Lateral Raise on Incline Bench	15-20	2	90
calves — Standing Calf Raise (two legs)	15-20	2	90
MODIFIED COMPOUND SUPERSET # 3 — biceps — Hammer Curl	15-20	2	90
triceps — Lying Dumbbell Extension	15-20	2	90
MODIFIED COMPOUND SUPERSET # 4 — thighs — Dumbbell Squat	15-20	2	90
hamstrings — Stiff-Legged Deadlift	15-20	2	90

Cardio and Abs

EXERCISE	TUESDAY/THURSDAY/SATURDAY		
	REPS	SETS	REST (seconds)
MODIFIED COMPOUND SUPERSET # 1 — abs — Lying Leg Raise	as many as you can	2	90
abs — Crunch	as many as you can	2	90

AEROBIC ACTIVITY

10 minutes of fast walking, stationary bike, or any other type of aerobic activity that you like. Don't be concerned at this stage with reaching the target heart rate; just concentrate on performing the activity at a comfortable but steady pace.

NOTES ON REPETITIONS

You will note that the repetition ranges are higher than what we normally recommend, which means using lighter weights. The reasons for this are the following:

* To start getting the joints and the muscles accustomed to weight training exercise while preventing injuries.
* To start creating neural pathways (links) between the brain and the muscles so that you start gaining better control and feel of the muscles in your body.

Please refer to www.BodySculptingBible.com for updated workouts and additional cardio routines.

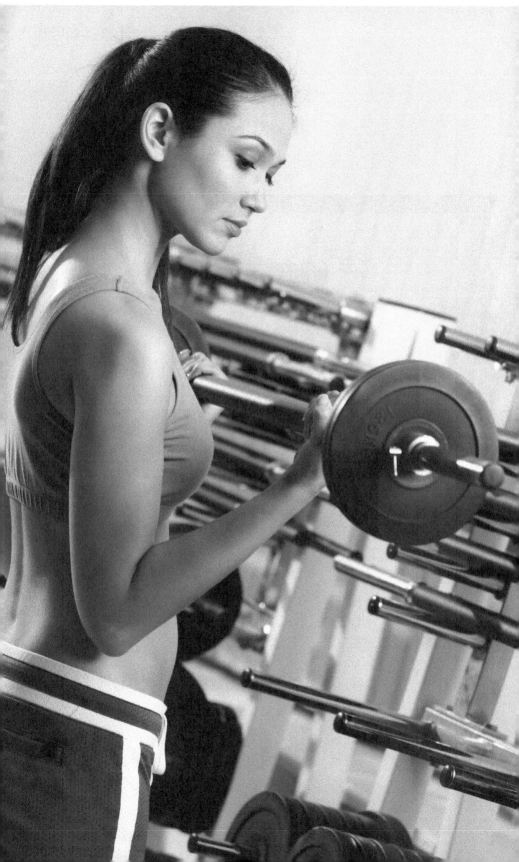

14-Day Body Sculpting Workout

14-DAY BODY SCULPTING WORKOUT

In this workout you will train with weights three days a week and perform aerobic activity three days a week. Sundays are your days off. You may choose to do Day 1 on Mondays, Day 2 on Wednesdays, and Day 3 on Fridays with Cardio and Abs on Tuesdays, Thursdays and Saturdays. Any other combination like Day 1 on Tuesdays, Day 2 on Thursdays, Day 3 on Saturdays, and Cardio with Abs on Wednesdays, Fridays and Sundays is also valid.

This workout is designed to be performed in the comfort of your home with minimum equipment, namely a pair of dumbbells or a pair of dumbbells with an adjustable bench. As you get stronger you may wish to purchase a pair of secure adjustable dumbbells such as Powerblocks.

14-Day Body Sculpting Workout

SPECIAL INSTRUCTIONS FOR WEEKS 1 & 2

Use modified compound supersets. Perform modified compound supersets by performing the first exercise, resting for the prescribed rest period, performing the second exercise, resting the prescribed rest period and going back to the first exercise. Continue in this manner until you have performed all of the prescribed number ofsets, and then continue with the next modified compound superset. You will repeat Day 1 on Monday, Day 2 on Wednesday, and Day 3 on Friday.

DAY 1

EXERCISE	REPS	SETS	REST (seconds)
Dumbbell One-Arm Row	12-15	2	90
Push-Up (against wall if unable to perform on floor)	12-15	2	90
Dumbbell Shoulder Press	12-15	2	90
Standing Calf Raise (one leg)	15-25	2	90
Dumbbell Curl	12-15	2	90
Overhead Dumbbell Extension	12-15	2	90
Dumbbell Squat	12-15	2	90
Stiff-Legged Deadlift	12-15	2	90

NOTES ON PUSH-UPS

Depending on your body weight, you may find this exercise difficult to do in the traditional way. If this is the case, then start by performing them standing against the wall (stand 1.5-2 ft. in front of the wall, extend your arms and perform the exercise). In this position you will not be lifting your full bodyweight. As you become stronger, you may perform push-ups against the floor "from your knees." Once you master that position, you will be able to perform the traditional push-up.

DAY 2

EXERCISE	REPS	SETS	REST (seconds)
Dumbbell Squat	12-15	2	90
Dumbbell Lunge	12-15	2	90
Ballet Squat	12-15	2	90
Stiff-Legged Deadlift	12-15	2	90
Standing Calf Raise (one leg)	15-25	2	90
Upright Row	12-15	2	90
Standing Calf Raise (two legs)	15-25	2	90
Triceps Kickback	12-15	2	90

Weeks 1 & 2

DAY 3		EXERCISE	REPS	SETS	REST (seconds)
					FRIDAY
MODIFIED COMPOUND SUPERSET #1	back	Two-Arm Row	12-15	2	90
	chest	Flat Dumbbell Fly (lying on the floor)	12-15	2	90
MODIFIED COMPOUND SUPERSET #2	shoulders	Bent-Over Lateral Raise on Incline Bench	12-15	2	90
	calves	Standing Calf Raise (two legs)	15-25	2	90
MODIFIED COMPOUND SUPERSET #3	biceps	Hammer Curl	12-15	2	90
	triceps	Lying Dumbbell Extension	12-15	2	90
MODIFIED COMPOUND SUPERSET #4	thighs	Ballet Squat	12-15	2	90
	hamstrings	Dumbbell Lunge	12-15	2	90

Cardio and Abs

		EXERCISE	REPS	SETS	REST (seconds)
					TUESDAY/THURSDAY/SATURDAY
MODIFIED COMPOUND SUPERSET #1	abs	Lying Leg Raise	as many as possible	2	90
	abs	Crunch	as many as possible	2	90

AEROBIC ACTIVITY
20 minutes of fast walking, stationary biking, or any other type of aerobic activity you enjoy while bringing you to your target heart rate.

Please refer to www.BodySculptingBible.com for updated workouts and additional cardio routines.

14-Day Body Sculpting Workout

SPECIAL INSTRUCTIONS FOR WEEKS 3 & 4

Use supersets. Perform supersets by pairing exercises with no rest period in between. Only rest after the two exercises have been performed consecutively. Repeat for the prescribed number of sets and then move on to the next pair of exercises. You will repeat Day 1 on Monday, Day 2 on Wednesday, and Day 3 on Friday.

DAY 1

EXERCISE		REPS	SETS	REST (seconds)
SUPERSET # 1	Dumbbell One-Arm Row	10-12	3	No Rest
	Push-Up (against wall if unable to perform on floor)	10-12	3	60
SUPERSET # 2	Dumbbell Shoulder Press	10-12	3	No Rest
	Standing Calf Raise (one leg)	15-25	3	60
SUPERSET # 3	Dumbbell Curl	10-12	3	No Rest
	Overhead Dumbbell Extension	10-12	3	60
SUPERSET # 4	Dumbbell Squat	10-12	3	No Rest
	Stiff-Legged Deadlift	10-12	3	60

NOTES ON PUSH-UPS

Depending on your body weight, you may find this exercise difficult to do in the traditional way. If this is the case, then start by performing them standing against the wall (stand 1.5-2 ft. in front of the wall, extend your arms and perform the exercise). In this position you will not be lifting your full bodyweight. As you become stronger, you may perform push-ups against the floor "from your knees." Once you master that position, you will be able to perform the traditional push-up.

DAY 2

EXERCISE		REPS	SETS	REST (seconds)
SUPERSET # 1	Dumbbell Squat	10-12	3	No Rest
	Dumbbell Lunge	10-12	3	60
SUPERSET # 2	Ballet Squat	10-12	3	No Rest
	Stiff-Legged Deadlift	10-12	3	60
SUPERSET # 3	Standing Calf Raise (one leg)	15-25	3	No Rest
	Upright Row	10-12	3	60
SUPERSET # 4	Standing Calf Raise (two legs)	15-25	3	No Rest
	Triceps Kickback	10-12	3	60

Weeks 3 & 4

DAY 3					FRIDAY
EXERCISE			**REPS**	**SETS**	**REST (seconds)**
SUPERSET # 1	back	Two-Arm Row	10-12	3	No Rest
	chest	Flat Dumbbell Fly (lying on the floor) (against wall if unable to perform on floor)	10-12	3	60
SUPERSET # 2	shoulders	Bent-Over Lateral Raise on Incline Bench	10-12	3	No Rest
	calves	Standing Calf Raise (two legs)	15-25	3	60
SUPERSET # 3	biceps	Hammer Curl	10-12	3	No Rest
	triceps	Lying Dumbbell Extension	10-12	3	60
SUPERSET # 4	thighs	Ballet Squat	10-12	3	No Rest
	hamstrings	Dumbbell Lunge	10-12	3	60

Cardio and Abs

					TUESDAY/THURSDAY/SATURDAY
EXERCISE			**REPS**	**SETS**	**REST (seconds)**
SUPERSET # 1	abs	Lying Leg Raise	as many as possible	3	No Rest
	abs	Crunch	as many as possible	3	60

AEROBIC ACTIVITY
30 minutes of fast walking, stationary biking, or any other type of aerobic activity you enjoy while bringing you to your target heart rate.

Please refer to www.BodySculptingBible.com for updated workouts and additional cardio routines.

14-Day Body Sculpting Workout

SPECIAL INSTRUCTIONS FOR WEEKS 5 & 6

Use giant sets. Perform giant sets by performing four exercises with no rest period in between. Only rest after the four exercises have been performed consecutively. Repeat for the prescribed number of sets and then move on to the second group of exercises. You will repeat Day 1 on Monday, Day 2 on Wednesday, and Day 3 on Friday.

DAY 1					MONDAY
EXERCISE			REPS	SETS	REST (seconds)
GIANT SET #1		Dumbbell Squat	8-10	4	No Rest
		Stiff-Legged Deadlift	8-10	4	No Rest
		Dumbbell One-Arm Row	8-10	4	No Rest
		Push-Up (against wall if unable to perform on floor)	8-10	4	60
GIANT SET #2		Dumbbell Shoulder Press	8-10	4	No Rest
		Standing Calf Raise (one leg)	15-25	4	No Rest
		Dumbbell Curl	8-10	4	No Rest
		Overhead Dumbbell Extension	8-10	4	60

NOTES ON PUSH-UPS

Depending on your body weight, you may find this exercise difficult to do in the traditional way. If this is the case, then start by performing them standing against the wall (stand 1.5-2 ft. in front of the wall, extend your arms and perform the exercise). In this position you will not be lifting your full bodyweight. As you become stronger, you may perform push-ups against the floor "from your knees." Once you master that position, you will be able to perform the traditional push-up.

DAY 2					WEDNESDAY
EXERCISE			REPS	SETS	REST (seconds)
GIANT SET #1		Dumbbell Squat	8-10	4	No Rest
		Dumbbell Lunge	8-10	4	No Rest
		Standing Calf Raise (one leg)	15-25	4	No Rest
		Upright Row	8-10	4	60
GIANT SET #2		Ballet Squat	8-10	4	No Rest
		Stiff-Legged Deadlift	8-10	4	No Rest
		Standing Calf Raise (two legs)	15-25	4	No Rest
		Triceps Kickback	8-10	4	60

Weeks 5 & 6

DAY 3					FRIDAY
EXERCISE			**REPS**	**SETS**	**REST (seconds)**
GIANT SET # 1	thighs	Ballet Squat	8-10	4	No Rest
	hamstrings	Dumbbell Lunge	8-10	4	No Rest
	back	Two-Arm Row	8-10	4	No Rest
	chest	Flat Dumbbell Fly (lying on the floor)	8-10	4	60
GIANT SET # 2	shoulders	Bent-Over Lateral Raise on Incline Bench	8-10	4	No Rest
	calves	Standing Calf Raise (two legs)	15-25	4	No Rest
	biceps	Hammer Curl	8-10	4	No Rest
	triceps	Lying Dumbbell Extension	8-10	4	60

Cardio and Abs

					TUESDAY/THURSDAY/SATURDAY
EXERCISE			**REPS**	**SETS**	**REST (seconds)**
GIANT SET # 1	abs	Lying Leg Raise	as many as possible	4	No Rest
	abs	Crunch	as many as possible	4	No Rest

AEROBIC ACTIVITY
40 minutes of fast walking, stationary biking, or any other type of aerobic activity that you enjoy while bringing you to your target heart rate.

Please refer to www.BodySculptingBible.com for updated workouts and additional cardio routines.

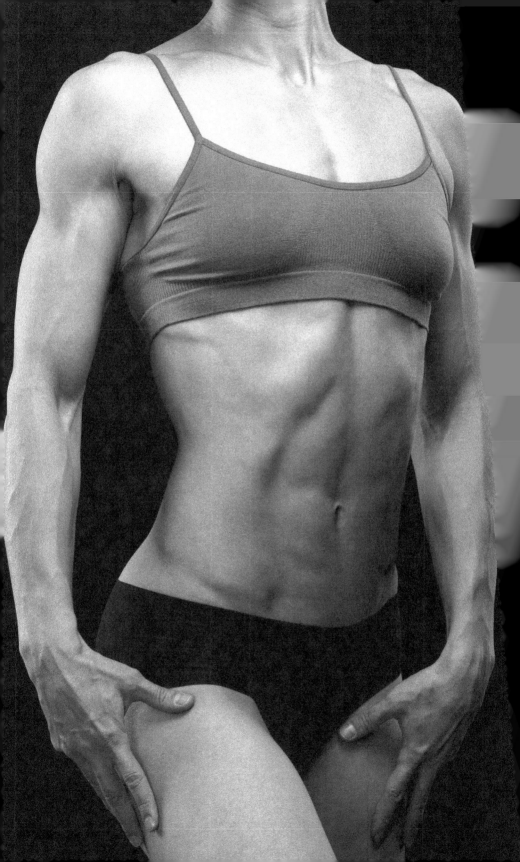

Advanced 14-Day Body Sculpting Workout

ADVANCED 14-DAY BODY SCULPTING WORKOUT

In this workout you will train with weights six days a week and perform aerobic activity six days a week. Sundays are your off days. You may do Day 1 on Mondays and Thursdays, Day 2 on Tuesdays and Fridays and Day 3 on Wednesdays and Saturdays.

This workout is designed to be performed at either a commercial gym or a very well equipped home gym. The reason for this is that we will be using a variety of exercises and training different angles and areas of the muscles in order to stimulate all muscle fibers.

Note that these routines provide alternate exercises. Alternate exercises are to be performed the next time that you perform the workout for that specific body part in order to provide varied stimulation. For example, if on Monday of week one you perform reverse curls as your first biceps exercise, on Friday you will perform preacher curls instead. This variation will help to avoid a plateau, keeping your muscle building capabilities in paramount shape.

Cardio and abs are to be performed on a daily basis preferably first thing in the morning on an empty stomach. The weight training workouts are to be performed in the afternoon or at any other convenient time. If your schedule does not allow for two separate sessions, then you may merge both sessions by performing the abs first, and then the weight training followed by the cardiovascular exercise.

Advanced 14-Day Body Sculpting Workout

SPECIAL INSTRUCTIONS FOR WEEKS 1 & 2

Use modified compound supersets. Perform the first exercise, resting for the prescribed rest period, perform the second exercise, rest the prescribed rest period and then go back to the first one. Continue in this manner until you have performed all of the prescribed number of sets. Then continue with the next modified compound superset.

DAY 1			MONDAY/THURSDAY
EXERCISE	**REPS**	**SETS**	**REST (seconds)**
Dumbbell One-Arm Row (alternate with Two-Arm Row,	12-15	3	90
Incline Dumbbell Press (alternate with palms facing each other grip)	12-15	3	90
Dumbbell Pullover (alternate with Seated Low-Pulley Row,	12-15	3	90
Chest Dip (alternate with Push-Up,	12-15	3	90
Wide Grip Pull-Up to Front (alternate with Straight Arm Pull-Down,	12-15	3	90
Incline Dumbbell Fly (alternate with Incline Cable Crossover,	12-15	3	90
Bent-Over Lateral Raise on Incline Bench (alternate with Seated Rear Delt Machine,	12-15	3	90
Seated Machine Calf Raise (alternate with Donkey Calf Raise,	15-25	3	90

DAY 2			
EXERCISE	**REPS**	**SETS**	**REST (seconds)**
Dumbbell Curl (alternate with Incline Dumbbell Curl,	12-15	3	90
Lying Dumbbell Extension (alternate with Triceps Pushdown,	12-15	3	90
Concentration Curl (alternate with Hammer Curl,	12-15	3	90
Triceps Kickback (alternate with Overhead Dumbbell Extension,	12-15	3	90
Reverse Curl (alternate with One-Arm Preacher Curl,	12-15	3	90
Triceps Dip (alternate with Close-Grip Dumbbell Press,	12-15	3	90
Dumbbell Shoulder Press (alternate with Military Press,	12-15	3	90
Upright Row (alternate with Dumbbell Lateral Raise,	12-15	3	90

Weeks 1 & 2

DAY 3			WEDNESDAY/SATURDAY	
EXERCISE		REPS	SETS	REST (seconds)
MODIFIED COMPOUND SUPERSET # 1 — thighs — Dumbbell Squat (alternate with Ballet Squat.	12-15	3	90
MODIFIED COMPOUND SUPERSET # 1 — hamstrings — Lying Leg Curl (alternate with Dumbbell Lunge.	12-15	3	90
MODIFIED COMPOUND SUPERSET # 2 — thighs — Hack Squat (alternate with Leg Extension,	12-15	3	90
MODIFIED COMPOUND SUPERSET # 2 — hamstrings — Stiff-Legged Deadlift (alternate with Seated Leg Curl Machine,	12-15	3	90
MODIFIED COMPOUND SUPERSET # 3 — thighs — Leg Press (alternate with Dumbbell Squat,	12-15	3	90
MODIFIED COMPOUND SUPERSET # 3 — hamstrings — Standing Hamstring Curl (alternate with Lying Leg Curl.	12-15	3	90
MODIFIED COMPOUND SUPERSET # 4 — calves — Calf Press (alternate with Multi-Directional Calf Raise,	15-25	3	90
MODIFIED COMPOUND SUPERSET # 4 — calves — Standing Calf Raise (one leg) (alternate with Standing Calf Raise (two legs),	15-25	3	90

Cardio and Abs

			ALL DAYS	
EXERCISE		REPS	SETS	REST (seconds)
MODIFIED COMPOUND SUPERSET # 1 — abs — Lying Leg Raise	15-25	3	90
MODIFIED COMPOUND SUPERSET # 1 — abs — Crunch	15-25	3	90
MODIFIED COMPOUND SUPERSET # 2 — abs — Knee-In	15-25	3	90
MODIFIED COMPOUND SUPERSET # 2 — abs — Incline Bench Partial Sit-Up	15-25	3	90

CARDIO AND ABS
To be performed from Monday through Saturday first thing in the morning on an empty stomach or right after the workout.

AEROBIC ACTIVITY
20 minutes of fast walking, stationary bike, or any other type of aerobic activity that you like at your target heart rate.

Please refer to www.BodySculptingBible.com for updated workouts and additional cardio routines.

Advanced 14-Day Body Sculpting Workout

SPECIAL INSTRUCTIONS FOR WEEKS 3 & 4

Use supersets. Perform supersets by pairing exercises with no rest period in between. Only rest after the two exercises have been performed consecutively. Repeat for the prescribed number of sets and then move on to the next pair of exercises. You will repeat Day 1 on Monday, Day 2 on Wednesday, and Day 3 on Friday.

DAY 1

EXERCISE	REPS	SETS	REST (seconds)
Dumbbell One-Arm Row (alternate with Two-Arm Row.	10-12	4	No Rest
Incline Dumbbell Press (alternate with palms facing each other grip)	10-12	4	60
Dumbbell Pullover (alternate with Seated Low-Pulley Row.	10-12	4	No Rest
Chest Dip (alternate with Push-Up.	10-12	4	60
Wide Grip Pull-Up to Front (alternate with Wide Grip Pull-Down.	10-12	3	No Rest
Incline Dumbbell Fly (alternate with Incline Cable Crossover.	10-12	3	60
Bent-Over Lateral Raise on Incline Bench (alternate with Seated Rear Delt Machine.	10-12	3	No Rest
Seated Machine Calf Raise (alternate with Donkey Calf Raise.	15-25	3	60

DAY 2

EXERCISE	REPS	SETS	REST (seconds)
Dumbbell Curl (alternate with Incline Dumbbell Curl.	10-12	4	No Rest
Lying Dumbbell Extension (alternate with Triceps Pushdown.	10-12	4	60
Concentration Curl (alternate with Hammer Curl.	10-12	4	No Rest
Triceps Kickback (alternate with Overhead Dumbbell Extension.	10-12	4	60
Reverse Curl (alternate with One-Arm Preacher Curl.	10-12	3	No Rest
Triceps Dip (alternate with Close-Grip Dumbbell Press.	10-12	3	60
Dumbbell Shoulder Press (alternate with Military Press.	10-12	3	No Rest
Upright Row (alternate with Dumbbell Lateral Raise.	10-12	3	60

Weeks 3 & 4

DAY 3				WEDNESDAY/SATURDAY
EXERCISE		REPS	SETS	REST (seconds)
SUPERSET # 1	thighs — Dumbbell Squat (alternate with Ballet Squat.	10-12	4	No Rest
	hamstrings — Lying Leg Curl (alternate with Dumbbell Lunge.	10-12	4	60
SUPERSET # 2	thighs — Hack Squat (alternate with Leg Extension.	10-12	4	No Rest
	hamstrings — Stiff-Legged Deadlift (alternate with Seated Leg Curl Machine.	10-12	4	60
SUPERSET # 3	thighs — Leg Press (alternate with Dumbbell Squat.	10-12	3	No Rest
	hamstrings — Standing Hamstring Curl (alternate with Lying Leg Curl.	10-12	3	60
SUPERSET # 4	calves — Calf Press (alternate with Multi-Directional Calf Raise.	15-25	3	No Rest
	calves — Standing Calf Raise (one leg) (alternate with Standing Calf Raise (two legs).	15-25	3	60

Cardio and Abs

				ALL DAYS
EXERCISE		REPS	SETS	REST (seconds)
SUPERSET # 1	abs — Lying Leg Raise	15-25	3	No Rest
	abs — Crunch	15-25	3	60
SUPERSET # 2	abs — Knee-In	15-25	3	No Rest
	abs — Incline Bench Partial Sit-Up	15-25	3	60

CARDIO AND ABS
To be performed from Monday through Saturday first thing in the morning on an empty stomach or right after the workout.

AEROBIC ACTIVITY
30 minutes of fast walking, stationary bike, or any other type of aerobic activity that you like at your target heart rate.

Please refer to www.BodySculptingBible.com for updated workouts and additional cardio routines.

Advanced 14-Day Body Sculpting Workout

SPECIAL INSTRUCTIONS FOR WEEKS 5 & 6

Use giant sets. Perform four exercises with no rest period in between. Only rest after the four exercises have been performed consecutively. Repeat for the prescribed number of sets and then move on to the second group of exercises.

DAY 1

	EXERCISE	REPS	SETS	REST (seconds)
GIANT SET #1	Dumbbell One-Arm Row (alternate with Two-Arm Row.	8-10	4	No Rest
	Incline Dumbbell Press (alternate with palms facing each other grip)	8-10	4	No Rest
	Dumbbell Pullover (alternate with Seated Low-Pulley Row.	8-10	4	No Rest
	Chest Dip (alternate with Push-Up,	8-10	4	60
GIANT SET #2	Wide Grip Pull-Up to Front (alternate with Straight Arm Pull-Down,	8-10	4	No Rest
	Incline Dumbbell Fly (alternate with Incline Cable Crossover,	8-10	4	No Rest
	Bent-Over Lateral Raise on Incline Bench (alternate with Seated Rear Delt Machine,	8-10	4	No Rest
	Seated Machine Calf Raise (alternate with Donkey Calf Raise.	15-25	4	60

DAY 2

	EXERCISE	REPS	SETS	REST (seconds)
GIANT SET #1	Dumbbell Curl (alternate with Incline Dumbbell Curl,	8-10	4	No Rest
	Lying Dumbbell Extension (alternate with Triceps Pushdown,	8-10	4	No Rest
	Concentration Curl (alternate with Hammer Curl,	8-10	4	No Rest
	Triceps Kickback (alternate with Overhead Dumbbell Extension,	8-10	4	60
GIANT SET #2	Reverse Curl (alternate with One-Arm Preacher Curl,	8-10	4	No Rest
	Triceps Dip (alternate with Close-Grip Dumbbell Press,	8-10	4	No Rest
	Dumbbell Shoulder Press (alternate with Military Press,	8-10	4	No Rest
	Upright Row (alternate with Dumbbell Lateral Raise,	8-10	4	60

Weeks 5 & 6

DAY 3				WEDNESDAY/SATURDAY	
EXERCISE		PAGE NO.	REPS	SETS	REST (seconds)
GIANT SET #1	Dumbbell Squat (alternate with Ballet Squat,		8-10	4	No Rest
	Lying Leg Curl (alternate with Dumbbell Lunge,		8-10	4	No Rest
	Hack Squat (alternate with Leg Extension,		8-10	4	No Rest
	Stiff-Legged Deadlift (alternate with Seated Leg Curl Machine,		8-10	4	60
GIANT SET #2	Leg Press (alternate with Dumbbell Squat,		8-10	4	No Rest
	Standing Hamstring Curl (alternate with Lying Leg Curl,		8-10	4	No Rest
	Calf Press (alternate with Multi-Directional Calf Raise,		8-10	4	No Rest
	Standing Calf Raise (one leg) (alternate with two legs.		8-10	4	60

Cardio and Abs

				ALL DAYS	
EXERCISE		PAGE NO.	REPS	SETS	REST (seconds)
GIANT SET #1	Lying Leg Raise		15-25	4	No Rest
	Crunch		15-25	4	No Rest
	Knee-In		15-25	4	No Rest
	Incline Bench Partial Sit-Up		15-25	4	60

CARDIO AND ABS
To be performed from Monday through Saturday first thing in the morning on an empty stomach or right after the workout.

AEROBIC ACTIVITY
40 minutes of fast walking, stationary bike, or any other type of aerobic activity that you like at your target heart rate.

WHAT TO DO AFTER WEEK SIX OF THE ADVANCED WORKOUT?

After week six, you can start over at week one but substitute the recommended exercises with similar ones. Don't be afraid to experiment! If you are satisfied with your lower body and want to equally emphasize the upper body, then you can adjust the routine to perform chest/back on Monday/Thursday, Shoulders and Arms on Tuesday/Friday, and Legs on Wednesday and Saturday.

Also, if you want to gain additional muscle mass, then feel free to reduce the amount of repetitions in the following manner:

Weeks 1-2: 10-12 reps
Weeks 3-4: 8-10 reps
Weeks 5-6: 6-8 reps

Also, reduce the cardiovascular/abs component of the workout to three days a week instead of six. All other aspects of the program remain the same.

(For more Body Sculpting workouts, please take a look at our book, *The Body Sculpting Bible for Women*.)

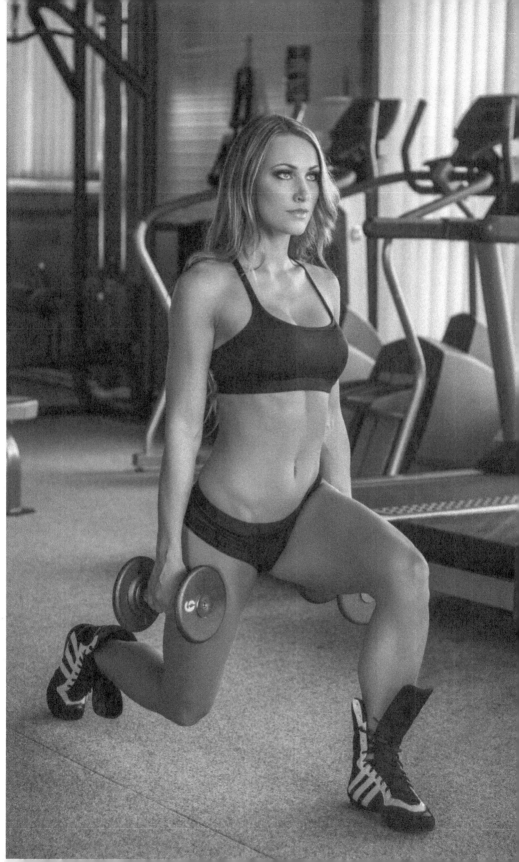

Buns and Legs Workout

Buns and Legs Workout

SPECIAL INSTRUCTIONS FOR WEEKS 1 & 2

Perform 12 to 15 repetitions of each exercise and two sets. Note that the pace of the workout is fast as well, in order to emphasize definition.

DAY 1			MONDAY
EXERCISE	**REPS**	**SETS**	**REST**
MODIFIED COMPOUND SUPERSET # 1			
Glutes and Quads: Dumbbell Squat	12–15	2	30 seconds
Glutes and Quads: Multi–Directional Lunges	12–15	2	30 seconds
Glutes and Quads: Leg Press on Machine	12–15	2	30 seconds
Glutes and Quads: One-Legged Butt Press with Ball	12–15	2	60 seconds
MODIFIED COMPOUND SUPERSET # 2			
Outer Thighs: Cable Leg Raise for Outer Thigh	12–15	2	30 seconds
Outer Thighs: Squat with Abduction	12–15	2	30 seconds
Inner Thighs: Wide Stance Squat	12–15	2	30 seconds
Inner Thighs: Ball Extension	12–15	2	60 seconds
AB WORKOUT			
Crunch on the Ball	20	3	30 seconds
Reverse Crunch with Legs Extended	20	3	30 seconds
Twist on the Ball	20	3	30 seconds
Crunch/Pelvic Lift Combination	20	3	30 seconds
Reverse Crunch	20	3	30 seconds
Lower Back Extension	20	3	30 seconds

Cardio: Follow with 20 minutes of cardiovascular exercise such as elliptical, stationary bike, treadmill, or any other activity that will raise your heart rate to at least (220 – (Your Age)) x 0.75 +/- 10 beats.

DAYS 2 AND 4	WEDNESDAY AND SATURDAY

On Wednesdays and Saturdays you can perform an upper body workout, such as the one presented in *The Body Sculpting Bible for Women*, followed by 20 minutes of cardiovascular exercise such as elliptical, stationary bike, treadmill, or any other activity that will raise your heart rate to at least (220 – (Your Age)) x 0.75 +/- 10 beats. For your upper body training, just follow the same repetition and rest schemes as the ones used for your lower body workouts.

Weeks 1 & 2

DAY 3			FRIDAY
EXERCISE	**REPS**	**SETS**	**REST**
MODIFIED COMPOUND SUPERSET # 1			
Glutes and Quads: One-Legged Squat	12–15	2	30 seconds
Glutes and Quads: Leg Extension Machine	12–15	2	30 seconds
Glutes and Quads: Ball Lunge	12–15	2	30 seconds
Glutes and Quads: Butt Blaster on Machine	12–15	2	60 seconds
MODIFIED COMPOUND SUPERSET #2			
Hamstrings: Hamstring Curl on the Ball	12–15	2	30 seconds
Hamstrings: Lying Hamstring Curl on Machine	12–15	2	30 seconds
Calves: Multi-Directional Calf Raises	12–15	2	30 seconds
Calves: Calf Press on Leg Press Machine	12–15	2	60 seconds
AB WORKOUT			
Crunch on the Ball	20	3	30 seconds
Reverse Crunch with Legs Extended	20	3	30 seconds
Twist on the Ball	20	3	30 seconds
Crunch/Pelvic Lift Combination	20	3	30 seconds
Reverse Crunch	20	3	30 seconds
Lower Back Extension	20	3	30 seconds

Cardio: Follow with 20 minutes of cardiovascular exercise such as elliptical, stationary bike, treadmill, or any other activity that will raise your heart rate to at least (220 – (Your Age)) x 0.75 +/– 10 beats.

Buns and Legs Workout

SPECIAL INSTRUCTIONS FOR WEEKS 3 & 4

Perform 10 to 12 repetitions of each exercise and three sets. Eliminate the rest in between some of the exercises as prescribed below.

DAY 1			MONDAY
EXERCISE	REPS	SETS	REST
SUPERSET # 1			
Glutes and Quads: Dumbbell Squat	10–12	3	0 seconds
Glutes and Quads: Multi–Directional Lunges	10–12	3	30 seconds
Glutes and Quads: Leg Press on Machine	10–12	3	0 seconds
Glutes and Quads: One-Legged Butt Press with Ball	10–12	3	60 seconds
SUPERSET # 2			
Outer Thighs: Cable Leg Raise for Outer Thigh	10–12	3	0 seconds
Outer Thighs: Squat with Abduction	10–12	3	30 seconds
Inner Thighs: Wide Stance Squat	10–12	3	0 seconds
Inner Thighs: Ball Extension	10–12	3	60 seconds
AB WORKOUT			
Crunch on the Ball	20	3	30 seconds
Reverse Crunch with Legs Extended	20	3	30 seconds
Twist on the Ball	20	3	30 seconds
Crunch/Pelvic Lift Combination	20	3	30 seconds
Reverse Crunch	20	3	30 seconds
Lower Back Extension	20	3	30 seconds

Cardio: Follow with 30 minutes of cardiovascular exercise such as elliptical, stationary bike, treadmill, or any other activity that will raise your heart rate to at least (220 – (Your Age)) x 0.75 +/– 10 beats.

DAYS 2 AND 4	WEDNESDAY AND SATURDAY

On Wednesdays and Saturdays you can perform an upper body workout, such as the one presented in *The Body Sculpting Bible for Women*, followed by 20 minutes of cardiovascular exercise such as elliptical, stationary bike, treadmill, or any other activity that will raise your heart rate to at least (220 – (Your Age)) x 0.75 +/– 10 beats. For your upper body training, just follow the same repetition and rest schemes as the ones used for your lower body workouts.

Weeks 3 & 4

DAY 3			FRIDAY
EXERCISE	**REPS**	**SETS**	**REST**
SUPERSET # 1			
Glutes and Quads: One-Legged Squat	10–12	3	0 seconds
Glutes and Quads: Leg Extension Machine	10–12	3	30 seconds
Glutes and Quads: Ball Lunge	10–12	3	0 seconds
Glutes and Quads: Butt Blaster on Machine	10–12	3	60 seconds
SUPERSET # 2			
Hamstrings: Hamstring Curl on the Ball	10–12	3	0 seconds
Hamstrings: Lying Hamstring Curl on Machine	10–12	3	30 seconds
Calves: Multi–Directional Calf Raises	10–12	3	0 seconds
Calves: Calf Press on Leg Press Machine	10–12	3	60 seconds
AB WORKOUT			
Crunch on the Ball	20	3	30 seconds
Reverse Crunch with Legs Extended	20	3	30 seconds
Twist on the Ball	20	3	30 seconds
Crunch/Pelvic Lift Combination	20	3	30 seconds
Reverse Crunch	20	3	30 seconds
Lower Back Extension	20	3	30 seconds

Cardio: Follow with 30 minutes of cardiovascular exercise such as elliptical, stationary bike, treadmill, or any other activity that will raise your heart rate to at least (220 – (Your Age)) x 0.75 +/– 10 beats.

Buns and Legs Workout

SPECIAL INSTRUCTIONS FOR WEEKS 5 & 6

Perform 8 to 10 repetitions of each exercise. Perform the exercises as Giant Sets, removing te rest period between exercises.

DAY 1			MONDAY
EXERCISE	REPS	SETS	REST
GIANT SET # 1			
Glutes and Quads: Dumbbell Squat	8–10	3	0 seconds
Glutes and Quads: Multi–Directional Lunges	8–10	3	0 seconds
Glutes and Quads: Leg Press on Machine	8–10	3	0 seconds
Glutes and Quads: One-Legged Butt Press with Ball	8–10	3	60 seconds
GIANT SET # 2			
Outer Thighs: Cable Leg Raise for Outer Thigh	8–10	3	0 seconds
Outer Thighs: Squat with Abduction	8–10	3	0 seconds
Inner Thighs: Wide Stance Squat	8–10	3	0 seconds
Inner Thighs: Ball Extension	8–10	3	60 seconds
AB WORKOUT			
Crunch on the Ball	20	3	30 seconds
Reverse Crunch with Legs Extended	20	3	30 seconds
Twist on the Ball	20	3	30 seconds
Crunch/Pelvic Lift Combination	20	3	30 seconds
Reverse Crunch	20	3	30 seconds
Lower Back Extension	20	3	30 seconds

Cardio: Follow with 40 minutes of cardiovascular exercise such as elliptical, stationary bike, treadmill, or any other activity that will raise your heart rate to at least (220 – (Your Age)) x 0.75 +/– 10 beats.

DAYS 2 AND 4	WEDNESDAY AND SATURDAY

On Wednesdays and Saturdays you can perform an upper body workout, such as the one presented in in *The Body Sculpting Bible for Women* followed by 40 minutes of cardiovascular exercise such as elliptical, stationary bike, treadmill, or any other activity that will raise your heart rate to at least (220 – (Your Age)) x 0.75 +/– 10 beats. For your upper body training, just follow the same repetition and rest schemes as the ones used for your lower body workouts.

Weeks 5 & 6

DAY 3			FRIDAY
EXERCISE	**REPS**	**SETS**	**REST**
GIANT SET # 1			
Glutes and Quads: One-Legged Squat	8–10	3	0 seconds
Glutes and Quads: Leg Extension Machine	8–10	3	0 seconds
Glutes and Quads: Ball Lunge	8–10	3	0 seconds
Glutes and Quads: Butt Blaster on Machine	8–10	3	60 seconds
GIANT SET # 2			
Hamstrings: Hamstring Curl on the Ball	8–10	3	0 seconds
Hamstrings: Lying Hamstring Curl on Machine	8–10	3	0 seconds
Calves: Multi-Directional Calf Raises	8–10	3	0 seconds
Calves: Calf Press on Leg Press Machine	8–10	3	60 seconds
AB WORKOUT			
Crunch on the Ball	20	3	30 seconds
Reverse Crunch with Legs Extended	20	3	30 seconds
Twist on the Ball	20	3	30 seconds
Crunch/Pelvic Lift Combination	20	3	30 seconds
Reverse Crunch	20	3	30 seconds
Lower Back Extension	20	3	30 seconds

Cardio: Follow with 40 minutes of cardiovascular exercise such as elliptical, stationary bike, treadmill, or any other activity that will raise your heart rate to at least (220 – (Your Age)) x 0.75 +/– 10 beats.

(For more workouts for the buns and legs, please take a look at our book, *The Body Sculpting Bible for Buns & Legs*.)

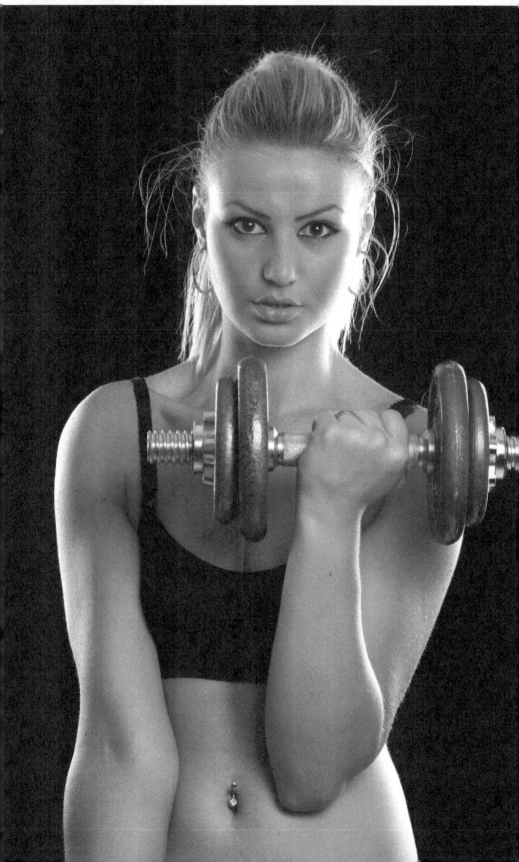

Express 21-Minute Workout

Express 21-Minute Workout

SPECIAL INSTRUCTIONS WEEKS 1 & 2

Use Modified Compound Supersets. Perform Modified Compound Supersets by doing the exercises and resting the prescribed amount of time until you have completed a circuit. Then start at the beginning and repeat for the recommended number of times before moving on to the next modified compound superset.

ABS AND CARDIO

EXERCISE	REPS	SETS	REST
MODIFIED COMPOUND SUPERSET # 1			
Lower Abs: Lying Leg Raises	12-15	2	30 seconds
Upper Abs: Crunches	12-15	2	30 seconds
Obliques: Bicycle	12-15	2	30 seconds
Aerobic Activity			
15 minutes of fast paced walking, stationary bike, or any other type of aerobic activity that you like.			

DAY 1

EXERCISE	REPS	SETS	REST
MODIFIED COMPOUND SUPERSET # 1			
Back: One-Arm Rows (Palms facing Torso)	12-15	2	30 seconds
Chest: Incline Dumbbell Bench Press	12-15	2	30 seconds
Thighs: Dumbbell Squats	12-15	2	30 seconds
Hamstrings: Dumbbell Stiff-Legged Deadlifts	12-15	2	30 seconds
MODIFIED COMPOUND SUPERSET # 2			
Biceps: Dumbbell Curls	12-15	2	30 seconds
Triceps: Lying Dumbbell Triceps Extensions	12-15	2	30 seconds
Shoulders: Dumbbell Upright Rows	12-15	2	30 seconds
Calves: Two-Legged Dumbbell Calf Raises	12-15	2	30 seconds

Weeks 1 & 2

DAY 2

EXERCISE	REPS	SETS	REST
MODIFIED COMPOUND SUPERSET # 1			
Thighs: Dumbbell Squats	12-15	2	30 seconds
Hamstrings: Static Dumbbell Lunges (Press with Heels)	12-15	2	30 seconds
Thighs: Wide-Stance Dumbbell Squats	12-15	2	30 seconds
Hamstrings: Dumbbell Stiff-Legged Deadlifts	12-15	2	30 seconds
MODIFIED COMPOUND SUPERSET # 2			
Calves: One-Legged Dumbbell Calf Raises	12-15	2	30 seconds
Shoulders: Bent-Over Lateral Raises	12-15	2	30 seconds
Calves: Two-Legged Dumbbell Calf Raises	12-15	2	30 seconds
Triceps: Lying Dumbbell Triceps Extension	12-15	2	30 seconds

DAY 3

EXERCISE	REPS	SETS	REST
FULL BODY COMBINATION WORKOUT # 1			
Back and Thighs: Squats with Dumbbell Rows	12-15	2	30 seconds
Chest and Core: Push-Ups with Side Rotation	12-15	2	30 seconds
Shoulders and Thighs: Upright Rows with Side-to-Side Lunges	12-15	2	30 seconds
Hamstrings and Back: Deadlift/Row Combo	12-15	2	30 seconds
FULL BODY COMBINATION WORKOUT # 2			
Biceps and Thighs: Knee-Ups into Back Lunge with Bicep Curl	12-15	2	30 seconds
Triceps and Thighs: Plié Squats with Triceps Extension	12-15	2	30 seconds
Shoulders and Thighs: Lunges with Overhead Press	12-15	2	30 seconds
Thighs: Squat with Alternating Leg Kick	12-15	2	30 seconds

Express 21-Minute Workout

SPECIAL INSTRUCTIONS WEEKS 3 & 4

Use Supersetting. Perform two exercises with no rest period in between. Rest for 30 seconds and then perform another two exercises with no rest in between. Repeat for the prescribed number of sets and then continue with the next group of exercises.

ABS AND CARDIO			
EXERCISE	REPS	SETS	REST
MODIFIED COMPOUND SUPERSET # 1			
Lower Abs: Lying Leg Raises	10-12	3	0 seconds
Upper Abs: Crunches	10-12	3	0 seconds
Obliques: Bicycle	10-12	2	30 seconds
Aerobic Activity			
15 minutes of fast paced walking, stationary bike, or any other type of aerobic activity that you like.			

DAY 1			
EXERCISE	REPS	SETS	REST
MODIFIED COMPOUND SUPERSET # 1			
Back: One-Arm Rows (Palms facing Torso)	10-12	3	0 seconds
Chest: Incline Dumbbell Bench Press	10-12	3	30 seconds
Thighs: Dumbbell Squats	10-12	3	0 seconds
Hamstrings: Dumbbell Stiff-Legged Deadlifts	10-12	3	30 seconds
MODIFIED COMPOUND SUPERSET # 2			
Biceps: Dumbbell Curls	10-12	3	0 seconds
Triceps: Lying Dumbbell Triceps Extensions	10-12	3	30 seconds
Shoulders: Dumbbell Upright Rows	10-12	3	0 seconds
Calves: Two-Legged Dumbbell Calf Raises	10-12	3	30 seconds

Weeks 3 & 4

DAY 2			
EXERCISE	**REPS**	**SETS**	**REST**
MODIFIED COMPOUND SUPERSET # 1			
Thighs: Dumbbell Squats	10-12	3	0 seconds
Hamstrings: Static Dumbbell Lunges (Press with Heels)	10-12	3	30 seconds
Thighs: Wide Stance Dumbbell Squats	10-12	3	0 seconds
Hamstrings: Dumbbell Stiff-Legged Deadlifts	10-12	3	30 seconds
MODIFIED COMPOUND SUPERSET # 2			
Calves: One-Legged Dumbbell Calf Raises	10-12	3	0 seconds
Shoulders: Bent-Over Lateral Raises	10-12	3	30 seconds
Calves: Two-Legged Dumbbell Calf Raises	10-12	3	0 seconds
Triceps: Lying Dumbbell Triceps Extension	10-12	3	30 seconds

DAY 3			
EXERCISE	**REPS**	**SETS**	**REST**
FULL BODY COMBINATION WORKOUT # 1			
Back and Thighs: Squats with Dumbbell Rows	10-12	3	0 seconds
Chest and Core: Push-Ups with Side Rotation	10-12	3	30 seconds
Shoulders and Thighs: Upright Rows with Side-to-Side Lunges	10-12	3	0 seconds
Hamstrings and Back: Deadlift/Row Combo	10-12	3	30 seconds
FULL BODY COMBINATION WORKOUT # 2			
Biceps and Thighs: Knee-Ups into Back Lunge with Bicep Curl	10-12	3	0 seconds
Triceps and Thighs: Plié Squats with Triceps Extension	10-12	3	30 seconds
Shoulders and Thighs: Lunges with Overhead Press	10-12	3	0 seconds
Thighs: Squat with Alternating Leg Kick	10-12	3	30 seconds

Express 21-Minute Workout

SPECIAL INSTRUCTIONS WEEKS 3 & 4

Use Giant Sets. Perform four exercises with no rest period in between. Only rest after the four exercises have been performed consecutively. Repeat for the prescribed number of sets and then continue with the next group of exercises.

ABS AND CARDIO			
EXERCISE	**REPS**	**SETS**	**REST**
GIANT SET # 1			
Lower Abs: Lying Leg Raises	8-10	3	0 seconds
Upper Abs: Crunches	8-10	3	0 seconds
Obliques: Bicycle	8-10	2	30 seconds
Aerobic Activity			
15 minutes of fast paced walking, stationary bike, or any other type of aerobic activity that you like.			

DAY 1			
EXERCISE	**REPS**	**SETS**	**REST**
GIANT SET # 1			
Back: One-Arm Rows (Palms facing Torso)	8-10	3	0 seconds
Chest: Incline Dumbbell Bench Press	8-10	3	0 seconds
Thighs: Dumbbell Squats	8-10	3	0 seconds
Hamstrings: Dumbbell Stiff-Legged Deadlifts	8-10	3	30 seconds
GIANT SET # 2			
Biceps: Dumbbell Curls	8-10	3	0 seconds
Triceps: Lying Dumbbell Triceps Extensions	8-10	3	0 seconds
Shoulders: Dumbbell Upright Rows	8-10	3	0 seconds
Calves: Two-Legged Dumbbell Calf Raises	8-10	3	30 seconds

Weeks 5 & 6

DAY 2			
EXERCISE	**REPS**	**SETS**	**REST**
GIANT SET # 1			
Thighs: Dumbbell Squats	8-10	3	0 seconds
Hamstrings: Static Dumbbell Lunges (Press with Heels)	8-10	3	0 seconds
Thighs: Wide-Stance Dumbbell Squats	8-10	3	0 seconds
Hamstrings: Dumbbell Stiff-Legged Deadlifts	8-10	3	30 seconds
GIANT SET # 2			
Calves: One-Legged Dumbbell Calf Raises	8-10	3	0 seconds
Shoulders: Bent-Over Lateral Raises	8-10	3	0 seconds
Calves: Two-Legged Dumbbell Calf Raises	8-10	3	0 seconds
Triceps: Lying Dumbbell Triceps Extension	8-10	3	30 seconds

DAY 3				
EXERCISE	**PAGE NO.**	**REPS**	**SETS**	**REST**
FULL BODY COMBINATION GIANT SET # 1 (HEAVIER WEIGHTS)				
Back and Thighs: Squats with Dumbbell Rows		8-10	3	0 seconds
Chest and Core: Push-Ups with Side Rotation		8-10	3	0 seconds
Shoulders and Thighs: Upright Rows with Side-to-Side Lunges		8-10	3	0 seconds
Hamstrings and Back: Deadlift/Row Combo		8-10	3	30 seconds
FULL BODY COMBINATION GIANT SET # 1 (HEAVIER WEIGHTS)				
Biceps and Thighs: Knee-Ups into Back Lunge with Bicep Curl		8-10	3	0 seconds
Triceps and Thighs: Plié Squats with Triceps Extension		8-10	3	0 seconds
Shoulders and Thighs: Lunges with Overhead Press		8-10	3	0 seconds
Thighs: Squat with Alternating Leg Kick		8-10	3	30 seconds

(For more express Body Sculpting workouts, please take a look at our book, *The Body Sculpting Bible Express for Women*.)

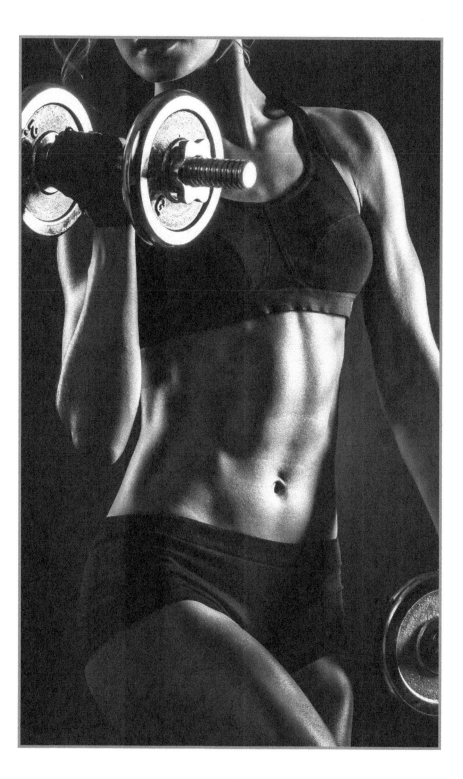

Part 2: Training Journal

DATE:_____

Daily Nutrition Journal

Week ⬤ Day ⬤

	Food	Serving Size	Calories	Carbs (grams)	Protein (grams)	Fat (grams)
Meal 1						
Meal 2						
Meal 3						
Meal 4						
Meal 5						
Meal 6						
Total						

DATE:_____

Daily Workout Journal Week ⬤ Day ⬤

	Exercise	Rest	Set 1 Reps	Weight	Set 2 Reps	Weight	Set 3 Reps	Weight	Set 4 Reps	Weight	Set 5 Reps	Weight
Group 1												
Group 2												
Group 3												
Group 4												
Abs												
Cardio	Cardio Activity: Average Heart Rate: Duration:	Notes:										

START TIME:_____   **END TIME:**_____

DATE:_____

Daily Nutrition Journal   Week ⬤   Day ⬤

	Food	Serving Size	Calories	Carbs (grams)	Protein (grams)	Fat (grams)
Meal 1						
Meal 2						
Meal 3						
Meal 4						
Meal 5						
Meal 6						
Total						

DATE:_____

Daily Workout Journal

Week ⬤ Day ⬤

Exercise	Rest	Set 1 Reps	Set 1 Weight	Set 2 Reps	Set 2 Weight	Set 3 Reps	Set 3 Weight	Set 4 Reps	Set 4 Weight	Set 5 Reps	Set 5 Weight
Group 1											
Group 2											
Group 3											
Group 4											
Abs											

Cardio

Cardio Activity: Notes:

Average Heart Rate:

Duration:

Notes

START TIME:_____   END TIME:_____

DATE:_____

Daily Nutrition Journal   Week ⬤   Day ⬤

	Food	Serving Size	Calories	Carbs (grams)	Protein (grams)	Fat (grams)
Meal 1						
Meal 2						
Meal 3						
Meal 4						
Meal 5						
Meal 6						
Total						

DATE:_____

Daily Workout Journal

Week ⬤ Day ⬤

Exercise	Rest	Set 1		Set 2		Set 3		Set 4		Set 5	
		Reps	Weight	Reps	Weight	Reps	Weight	Reps	Weight	Reps	Weight
Group 1											
Group 2											
Group 3											
Group 4											
Abs											

Cardio

Cardio Activity: Notes: **Notes**

Average Heart Rate:

Duration:

START TIME:_____   END TIME:_____

DATE:_____

Daily Nutrition Journal   Week ⬤   Day ⬤

	Food	Serving Size	Calories	Carbs (grams)	Protein (grams)	Fat (grams)	
Meal 1							Meal 1
Meal 2							Meal 2
Meal 3							Meal 3
Meal 4							Meal 4
Meal 5							Meal 5
Meal 6							Meal 6
	Total						

DATE:_____

Daily Workout Journal

Week ◯ Day ◯

	Exercise	Rest	Set 1 Reps	Set 1 Weight	Set 2 Reps	Set 2 Weight	Set 3 Reps	Set 3 Weight	Set 4 Reps	Set 4 Weight	Set 5 Reps	Set 5 Weight	
Group 1													**Group 1**
Group 2													**Group 2**
Group 3													**Group 3**
Group 4													**Group 4**
Abs													**Abs**

Cardio | Cardio Activity: Notes: | **Notes**
Average Heart Rate:
Duration:

START TIME:_____   **END TIME:**_____

DATE:_____

Daily Nutrition Journal

Week ◯ Day ◯

	Food	Serving Size	Calories	Carbs (grams)	Protein (grams)	Fat (grams)
Meal 1						
Meal 2						
Meal 3						
Meal 4						
Meal 5						
Meal 6						
Total						

DATE:_____

Daily Workout Journal   Week ⬤   Day ⬤

Exercise	Rest	Set 1		Set 2		Set 3		Set 4		Set 5	
		Reps	Weight	Reps	Weight	Reps	Weight	Reps	Weight	Reps	Weight
Group 1											
Group 2											
Group 3											
Group 4											
Abs											

Cardio

Cardio Activity: Notes:

Average Heart Rate:

Duration:

START TIME:_____   **END TIME:**_____

DATE:_____

Daily Nutrition Journal   Week ⬤   Day ⬤

	Food	Serving Size	Calories	Carbs (grams)	Protein (grams)	Fat (grams)
Meal 1						
Meal 2						
Meal 3						
Meal 4						
Meal 5						
Meal 6						
Total						

DATE:_____

Daily Workout Journal

Week ⚪ Day ⚪

	Exercise	Rest	Set 1 Reps	Set 1 Weight	Set 2 Reps	Set 2 Weight	Set 3 Reps	Set 3 Weight	Set 4 Reps	Set 4 Weight	Set 5 Reps	Set 5 Weight	
Group 1													**Group 1**
Group 2													**Group 2**
Group 3													**Group 3**
Group 4													**Group 4**
Abs													**Abs**
Cardio	Cardio Activity:				Notes:								**Notes**
	Average Heart Rate:												
	Duration:												

START TIME:_____   **END TIME:**_____

DATE:_____

Daily Nutrition Journal   Week ●   Day ●

	Food	Serving Size	Calories	Carbs (grams)	Protein (grams)	Fat (grams)
Meal 1						
Meal 2						
Meal 3						
Meal 4						
Meal 5						
Meal 6						
Total						

DATE:_____

Daily Workout Journal

Week ◯ Day ◯

Exercise	Rest	Set 1		Set 2		Set 3		Set 4		Set 5	
		Reps	Weight	Reps	Weight	Reps	Weight	Reps	Weight	Reps	Weight
Group 1											
Group 2											
Group 3											
Group 4											
Abs											

Cardio

Cardio Activity: Notes:

Average Heart Rate:

Duration:

START TIME:_____   END TIME:_____

DATE:_____

Daily Nutrition Journal

Week ⬤ Day ⬤

	Food	Serving Size	Calories	Carbs (grams)	Protein (grams)	Fat (grams)
Meal 1						
Meal 2						
Meal 3						
Meal 4						
Meal 5						
Meal 6						
Total						

DATE:_____

Daily Workout Journal

Week ⬤   Day ⬤

	Exercise	Rest	Set 1		Set 2		Set 3		Set 4		Set 5	
			Reps	Weight	Reps	Weight	Reps	Weight	Reps	Weight	Reps	Weight
Group 1												
Group 2												
Group 3												
Group 4												
Abs												

Cardio Activity: Notes:

Average Heart Rate:

Duration:

START TIME:_____   END TIME:_____

DATE:_____

Daily Nutrition Journal

Week ⦿   Day ⦿

	Food	Serving Size	Calories	Carbs (grams)	Protein (grams)	Fat (grams)
Meal 1						
Meal 2						
Meal 3						
Meal 4						
Meal 5						
Meal 6						
Total						

DATE:_____

Daily Workout Journal

Week ◯ Day ◯

Exercise	Rest	Set 1		Set 2		Set 3		Set 4		Set 5	
		Reps	Weight	Reps	Weight	Reps	Weight	Reps	Weight	Reps	Weight
Group 1											
Group 2											
Group 3											
Group 4											
Abs											

Cardio

Cardio Activity: Notes:

Average Heart Rate:

Duration:

START TIME:_____   END TIME:_____

DATE:_____

Daily Nutrition Journal

Week ●   Day ●

	Food	Serving Size	Calories	Carbs (grams)	Protein (grams)	Fat (grams)
Meal 1						
Meal 2						
Meal 3						
Meal 4						
Meal 5						
Meal 6						
Total						

DATE:_____

Daily Workout Journal

Week ⬤   Day ⬤

	Exercise	Rest	Set 1 Reps	Weight	Set 2 Reps	Weight	Set 3 Reps	Weight	Set 4 Reps	Weight	Set 5 Reps	Weight
Group 1												
Group 2												
Group 3												
Group 4												
Abs												

Cardio

Cardio Activity: Notes:

Average Heart Rate:

Duration:

START TIME:_____   **END TIME:**_____

DATE:_____

Daily Nutrition Journal   Week ⚪   Day ⚪

	Food	Serving Size	Calories	Carbs (grams)	Protein (grams)	Fat (grams)
Meal 1						
Meal 2						
Meal 3						
Meal 4						
Meal 5						
Meal 6						
Total						

DATE:_____

Daily Workout Journal   Week ●   Day ●

	Exercise	Rest	Set 1 Reps	Weight	Set 2 Reps	Weight	Set 3 Reps	Weight	Set 4 Reps	Weight	Set 5 Reps	Weight	
Group 1													**Group 1**
Group 2													**Group 2**
Group 3													**Group 3**
Group 4													**Group 4**
Abs													**Abs**
Cardio	Cardio Activity: Notes: Average Heart Rate: Duration:												**Notes**

START TIME:_____   **END TIME:**_____

DATE:_____

Daily Nutrition Journal   Week ⬤   Day ⬤

	Food	Serving Size	Calories	Carbs (grams)	Protein (grams)	Fat (grams)
Meal 1						
Meal 2						
Meal 3						
Meal 4						
Meal 5						
Meal 6						
Total						

DATE:_____

Daily Workout Journal

Week ● Day ●

Exercise	Rest	Set 1 Reps	Weight	Set 2 Reps	Weight	Set 3 Reps	Weight	Set 4 Reps	Weight	Set 5 Reps	Weight
Group 1											
Group 2											
Group 3											
Group 4											
Abs											

Cardio

Cardio Activity:

Average Heart Rate:

Duration:

Notes

Notes:

START TIME:_____ **END TIME:**_____

DATE:_____

Daily Nutrition Journal   Week ⬤   Day ⬤

	Food	Serving Size	Calories	Carbs (grams)	Protein (grams)	Fat (grams)
Meal 1						
Meal 2						
Meal 3						
Meal 4						
Meal 5						
Meal 6						
Total						

DATE:_____

Daily Workout Journal   Week ⬤   Day ⬤

	Exercise	Rest	Set 1 Reps	Set 1 Weight	Set 2 Reps	Set 2 Weight	Set 3 Reps	Set 3 Weight	Set 4 Reps	Set 4 Weight	Set 5 Reps	Set 5 Weight
Group 1												
Group 2												
Group 3												
Group 4												
Abs												

Cardio	Cardio Activity:	Notes:	Notes
	Average Heart Rate:		
	Duration:		

START TIME:_____   END TIME:_____

DATE:_____

Daily Nutrition Journal

Week ⬤　　Day ⬤

	Food	Serving Size	Calories	Carbs (grams)	Protein (grams)	Fat (grams)
Meal 1						
Meal 2						
Meal 3						
Meal 4						
Meal 5						
Meal 6						
Total						

DATE:_____

Daily Workout Journal

Week ● Day ●

	Exercise	Rest	Set 1		Set 2		Set 3		Set 4		Set 5	
			Reps	Weight	Reps	Weight	Reps	Weight	Reps	Weight	Reps	Weight
Group 1												
Group 2												
Group 3												
Group 4												
Abs												

Cardio

Cardio Activity:

Average Heart Rate:

Duration:

Notes:

START TIME:_____   END TIME:_____

DATE:_____

Daily Nutrition Journal   Week ⬤   Day ⬤

	Food	Serving Size	Calories	Carbs (grams)	Protein (grams)	Fat (grams)
Meal 1						
Meal 2						
Meal 3						
Meal 4						
Meal 5						
Meal 6						
Total						

DATE:_____

Daily Workout Journal   Week ⬤   Day ⬤

Exercise	Rest	Set 1		Set 2		Set 3		Set 4		Set 5	
		Reps	Weight	Reps	Weight	Reps	Weight	Reps	Weight	Reps	Weight
Group 1											
Group 2											
Group 3											
Group 4											
Abs											

Cardio

Cardio Activity: Notes:

Average Heart Rate:

Duration:

START TIME:_____   **END TIME:**_____

DATE:_____

Daily Nutrition Journal   Week ⬤   Day ⬤

	Food	Serving Size	Calories	Carbs (grams)	Protein (grams)	Fat (grams)
Meal 1						
Meal 2						
Meal 3						
Meal 4						
Meal 5						
Meal 6						
Total						

DATE:_____

Daily Workout Journal   Week ⬤   Day ⬤

Exercise	Rest	Set 1 Reps	Weight	Set 2 Reps	Weight	Set 3 Reps	Weight	Set 4 Reps	Weight	Set 5 Reps	Weight
Group 1											
Group 2											
Group 3											
Group 4											
Abs											

Cardio

Cardio Activity: Notes:

Average Heart Rate:

Duration:

START TIME:_____   **END TIME:**_____

DATE:_____

Daily Nutrition Journal   Week ⬤   Day ⬤

	Food	Serving Size	Calories	Carbs (grams)	Protein (grams)	Fat (grams)
Meal 1						
Meal 2						
Meal 3						
Meal 4						
Meal 5						
Meal 6						
Total						

DATE:_____

Daily Workout Journal   Week ⬤   Day ⬤

	Exercise	Rest	Set 1 Reps	Weight	Set 2 Reps	Weight	Set 3 Reps	Weight	Set 4 Reps	Weight	Set 5 Reps	Weight
Group 1												
Group 2												
Group 3												
Group 4												
Abs												

Cardio / **Notes**

Cardio Activity: Notes:
Average Heart Rate:
Duration:

START TIME:_____   END TIME:_____

DATE:_____

Daily Nutrition Journal

Week ●   Day ●

	Food	Serving Size	Calories	Carbs (grams)	Protein (grams)	Fat (grams)
Meal 1						
Meal 2						
Meal 3						
Meal 4						
Meal 5						
Meal 6						
Total						

DATE:_____

Daily Workout Journal

Week ⬤   Day ⬤

	Exercise	Rest	Set 1 Reps	Weight	Set 2 Reps	Weight	Set 3 Reps	Weight	Set 4 Reps	Weight	Set 5 Reps	Weight	
Group 1													**Group 1**
Group 2													**Group 2**
Group 3													**Group 3**
Group 4													**Group 4**
Abs													**Abs**

Cardio	Cardio Activity: Notes:	**Notes**
	Average Heart Rate:	
	Duration:	

START TIME:_____   **END TIME:**_____

DATE:_____

Daily Nutrition Journal   Week ◯   Day ◯

	Food	Serving Size	Calories	Carbs (grams)	Protein (grams)	Fat (grams)
Meal 1						
Meal 2						
Meal 3						
Meal 4						
Meal 5						
Meal 6						
Total						

DATE:_____

Daily Workout Journal   Week ⚪   Day ⚪

	Exercise	Rest	Set 1 Reps	Set 1 Weight	Set 2 Reps	Set 2 Weight	Set 3 Reps	Set 3 Weight	Set 4 Reps	Set 4 Weight	Set 5 Reps	Set 5 Weight	
Group 1													**Group 1**
Group 2													**Group 2**
Group 3													**Group 3**
Group 4													**Group 4**
Abs													**Abs**
Cardio	Cardio Activity: Notes: Average Heart Rate: Duration:												**Notes**

START TIME:_____   **END TIME:**_____

DATE:_____

Daily Nutrition Journal

Week ●   Day ●

	Food	Serving Size	Calories	Carbs (grams)	Protein (grams)	Fat (grams)
Meal 1						
Meal 2						
Meal 3						
Meal 4						
Meal 5						
Meal 6						
Total						

DATE:_____

Daily Workout Journal

Week ◯ Day ◯

	Exercise	Rest	Set 1 Reps	Set 1 Weight	Set 2 Reps	Set 2 Weight	Set 3 Reps	Set 3 Weight	Set 4 Reps	Set 4 Weight	Set 5 Reps	Set 5 Weight	
Group 1													Group 1
Group 2													Group 2
Group 3													Group 3
Group 4													Group 4
Abs													Abs

Cardio	Cardio Activity: Notes: Average Heart Rate: Duration:	Notes

START TIME:_____   **END TIME:**_____

DATE:_____

Daily Nutrition Journal   Week ◯   Day ◯

	Food	Serving Size	Calories	Carbs (grams)	Protein (grams)	Fat (grams)
Meal 1						
Meal 2						
Meal 3						
Meal 4						
Meal 5						
Meal 6						
Total						

DATE:_____

Daily Workout Journal

Week ⬤ Day ⬤

Exercise	Rest	Set 1 Reps	Set 1 Weight	Set 2 Reps	Set 2 Weight	Set 3 Reps	Set 3 Weight	Set 4 Reps	Set 4 Weight	Set 5 Reps	Set 5 Weight
Group 1											
Group 2											
Group 3											
Group 4											
Abs											

Cardio Activity: Notes:

Average Heart Rate:

Duration:

START TIME:_____   END TIME:_____

DATE:_____

Daily Nutrition Journal   Week ⬤   Day ⬤

	Food	Serving Size	Calories	Carbs (grams)	Protein (grams)	Fat (grams)
Meal 1						
Meal 2						
Meal 3						
Meal 4						
Meal 5						
Meal 6						
Total						

DATE:_____

Daily Workout Journal

Week ⬤ Day ⬤

	Exercise	Rest	Set 1 Reps	Set 1 Weight	Set 2 Reps	Set 2 Weight	Set 3 Reps	Set 3 Weight	Set 4 Reps	Set 4 Weight	Set 5 Reps	Set 5 Weight	
Group 1													**Group 1**
Group 2													**Group 2**
Group 3													**Group 3**
Group 4													**Group 4**
Abs													**Abs**

Cardio	Cardio Activity: Average Heart Rate: Duration:	Notes:	**Notes**

START TIME:_____   END TIME:_____

DATE:_____

Daily Nutrition Journal   Week ⬤   Day ⬤

	Food	Serving Size	Calories	Carbs (grams)	Protein (grams)	Fat (grams)
Meal 1						
Meal 2						
Meal 3						
Meal 4						
Meal 5						
Meal 6						
	Total					

DATE:_____

Daily Workout Journal

Week ⦿   Day ⦿

Exercise	Rest	Set 1 Reps	Weight	Set 2 Reps	Weight	Set 3 Reps	Weight	Set 4 Reps	Weight	Set 5 Reps	Weight
Group 1											
Group 2											
Group 3											
Group 4											
Abs											

Cardio

Cardio Activity: Notes:

Average Heart Rate:

Duration:

START TIME:_____   **END TIME:**_____

DATE:_____

Daily Nutrition Journal   Week ⬤   Day ⬤

	Food	Serving Size	Calories	Carbs (grams)	Protein (grams)	Fat (grams)
Meal 1						
Meal 2						
Meal 3						
Meal 4						
Meal 5						
Meal 6						
Total						

DATE:_____

Daily Workout Journal

Week ○   Day ○

Exercise	Rest	Set 1 Reps	Weight	Set 2 Reps	Weight	Set 3 Reps	Weight	Set 4 Reps	Weight	Set 5 Reps	Weight
Group 1											
Group 2											
Group 3											
Group 4											
Abs											

Cardio

Cardio Activity: Notes:

Average Heart Rate:

Duration:

Notes

START TIME:_____   **END TIME:_____**

DATE:_____

Daily Nutrition Journal

Week ● Day ●

	Food	Serving Size	Calories	Carbs (grams)	Protein (grams)	Fat (grams)
Meal 1						
Meal 2						
Meal 3						
Meal 4						
Meal 5						
Meal 6						
Total						

DATE:_____

Daily Workout Journal

Week ⬤ Day ⬤

Exercise	Rest	Set 1		Set 2		Set 3		Set 4		Set 5	
		Reps	Weight	Reps	Weight	Reps	Weight	Reps	Weight	Reps	Weight
Group 1											
Group 2											
Group 3											
Group 4											
Abs											

Cardio

Cardio Activity:

Average Heart Rate:

Duration:

Notes:

START TIME:_____   END TIME:_____

DATE:_____

Daily Nutrition Journal   Week ⬤   Day ⬤

	Food	Serving Size	Calories	Carbs (grams)	Protein (grams)	Fat (grams)
Meal 1						
Meal 2						
Meal 3						
Meal 4						
Meal 5						
Meal 6						
Total						

DATE:_____

Daily Workout Journal

Week ⬤ Day ⬤

	Exercise	Rest	Set 1		Set 2		Set 3		Set 4		Set 5	
			Reps	Weight	Reps	Weight	Reps	Weight	Reps	Weight	Reps	Weight
Group 1												
Group 2												
Group 3												
Group 4												
Abs												

Cardio
Cardio Activity: Notes:
Average Heart Rate:
Duration:

Notes

START TIME:_____   END TIME:_____

DATE:_____

Daily Nutrition Journal   Week ◯   Day ◯

	Food	Serving Size	Calories	Carbs (grams)	Protein (grams)	Fat (grams)
Meal 1						
Meal 2						
Meal 3						
Meal 4						
Meal 5						
Meal 6						
Total						

DATE:_____

Daily Workout Journal   Week ⚪   Day ⚪

	Exercise	Rest	Set 1		Set 2		Set 3		Set 4		Set 5	
			Reps	Weight	Reps	Weight	Reps	Weight	Reps	Weight	Reps	Weight
Group 1												
Group 2												
Group 3												
Group 4												
Abs												
Cardio	Cardio Activity: Notes: Average Heart Rate: Duration:											

START TIME:_____   **END TIME:**_____

DATE:_____

Daily Nutrition Journal

Week ⚪   Day ⚪

	Food	Serving Size	Calories	Carbs (grams)	Protein (grams)	Fat (grams)
Meal 1						
Meal 2						
Meal 3						
Meal 4						
Meal 5						
Meal 6						
Total						

DATE:_____

Daily Workout Journal   Week ⬤   Day ⬤

	Exercise	Rest	Set 1 Reps	Weight	Set 2 Reps	Weight	Set 3 Reps	Weight	Set 4 Reps	Weight	Set 5 Reps	Weight	
Group 1													**Group 1**
Group 2													**Group 2**
Group 3													**Group 3**
Group 4													**Group 4**
Abs													**Abs**

Cardio

Cardio Activity: Notes:

Average Heart Rate:

Duration:

Notes

START TIME:_____   **END TIME:**_____

DATE:_____

Daily Nutrition Journal

Week ⬤ Day ⬤

	Food	Serving Size	Calories	Carbs (grams)	Protein (grams)	Fat (grams)
Meal 1						
Meal 2						
Meal 3						
Meal 4						
Meal 5						
Meal 6						
Total						

DATE:_____

Daily Workout Journal   Week ⬤   Day ⬤

	Exercise	Rest	Set 1 Reps	Set 1 Weight	Set 2 Reps	Set 2 Weight	Set 3 Reps	Set 3 Weight	Set 4 Reps	Set 4 Weight	Set 5 Reps	Set 5 Weight	
Group 1													**Group 1**
Group 2													**Group 2**
Group 3													**Group 3**
Group 4													**Group 4**
Abs													**Abs**

Cardio	Cardio Activity: Notes:	**Notes**
	Average Heart Rate:	
	Duration:	

START TIME:_____   **END TIME:**_____

DATE:_____

Daily Nutrition Journal   Week ⬤   Day ⬤

	Food	Serving Size	Calories	Carbs (grams)	Protein (grams)	Fat (grams)
Meal 1						
Meal 2						
Meal 3						
Meal 4						
Meal 5						
Meal 6						
Total						

DATE:_____

Daily Workout Journal

Week ○　　Day ○

	Exercise	Rest	Set 1 Reps	Set 1 Weight	Set 2 Reps	Set 2 Weight	Set 3 Reps	Set 3 Weight	Set 4 Reps	Set 4 Weight	Set 5 Reps	Set 5 Weight	
Group 1													**Group 1**
Group 2													**Group 2**
Group 3													**Group 3**
Group 4													**Group 4**
Abs													**Abs**
Cardio	Cardio Activity:　　　Notes: Average Heart Rate: Duration:												**Notes**

START TIME:_____　　　**END TIME:**_____

DATE:_____

Daily Nutrition Journal   Week ⬤   Day ⬤

	Food	Serving Size	Calories	Carbs (grams)	Protein (grams)	Fat (grams)
Meal 1						
Meal 2						
Meal 3						
Meal 4						
Meal 5						
Meal 6						
Total						

DATE:_____

Daily Workout Journal   Week ⬤   Day ⬤

Exercise	Rest	Set 1 Reps	Set 1 Weight	Set 2 Reps	Set 2 Weight	Set 3 Reps	Set 3 Weight	Set 4 Reps	Set 4 Weight	Set 5 Reps	Set 5 Weight
Group 1											
Group 2											
Group 3											
Group 4											
Abs											

Cardio

Cardio Activity: Notes:

Average Heart Rate:

Duration:

START TIME:_____   **END TIME:**_____

DATE:_____

Daily Nutrition Journal   Week ●   Day ●

	Food	Serving Size	Calories	Carbs (grams)	Protein (grams)	Fat (grams)
Meal 1						
Meal 2						
Meal 3						
Meal 4						
Meal 5						
Meal 6						
Total						

DATE:_____

Daily Workout Journal   Week ⬤   Day ⬤

Exercise	Rest	Set 1		Set 2		Set 3		Set 4		Set 5	
		Reps	Weight	Reps	Weight	Reps	Weight	Reps	Weight	Reps	Weight
Group 1											
Group 2											
Group 3											
Group 4											
Abs											

Cardio

Cardio Activity: Notes:

Average Heart Rate:

Duration:

START TIME:_____   **END TIME:**_____

DATE:_____

Daily Nutrition Journal Week ⬤ Day ⬤

	Food	Serving Size	Calories	Carbs (grams)	Protein (grams)	Fat (grams)
Meal 1						
Meal 2						
Meal 3						
Meal 4						
Meal 5						
Meal 6						
Total						

DATE:_____

Daily Workout Journal   Week ⚪   Day ⚪

Exercise	Rest	Set 1		Set 2		Set 3		Set 4		Set 5	
		Reps	Weight	Reps	Weight	Reps	Weight	Reps	Weight	Reps	Weight
Group 1											
Group 2											
Group 3											
Group 4											
Abs											

Cardio

Cardio Activity: Notes:

Average Heart Rate:

Duration:

START TIME:_____   **END TIME:**_____

DATE:_____

Daily Nutrition Journal   Week ○   Day ○

	Food	Serving Size	Calories	Carbs (grams)	Protein (grams)	Fat (grams)
Meal 1						
Meal 2						
Meal 3						
Meal 4						
Meal 5						
Meal 6						
Total						

DATE:_____

Daily Workout Journal

Week ● Day ●

	Exercise	Rest	Set 1 Reps	Weight	Set 2 Reps	Weight	Set 3 Reps	Weight	Set 4 Reps	Weight	Set 5 Reps	Weight	
Group 1													**Group 1**
Group 2													**Group 2**
Group 3													**Group 3**
Group 4													**Group 4**
Abs													**Abs**
Cardio	Cardio Activity:			Notes:									**Notes**
	Average Heart Rate:												
	Duration:												

START TIME:_____   END TIME:_____

DATE:_____

Daily Nutrition Journal

Week ⬤   Day ⬤

	Food	Serving Size	Calories	Carbs (grams)	Protein (grams)	Fat (grams)
Meal 1						
Meal 2						
Meal 3						
Meal 4						
Meal 5						
Meal 6						
Total						

DATE:_____

Daily Workout Journal   Week ⬤   Day ⬤

	Exercise	Rest	Set 1		Set 2		Set 3		Set 4		Set 5	
			Reps	Weight	Reps	Weight	Reps	Weight	Reps	Weight	Reps	Weight
Group 1												
Group 2												
Group 3												
Group 4												
Abs												
Cardio	Cardio Activity: Average Heart Rate: Duration:			Notes:								

Group 1 · Group 2 · Group 3 · Group 4 · Abs · Notes

START TIME:_____   END TIME:_____

DATE:_____

Daily Nutrition Journal   Week ⬤   Day ⬤

	Food	Serving Size	Calories	Carbs (grams)	Protein (grams)	Fat (grams)
Meal 1						
Meal 2						
Meal 3						
Meal 4						
Meal 5						
Meal 6						
Total						

DATE:_____

Daily Workout Journal

Week ⚪ Day ⚪

Exercise	Rest	Set 1		Set 2		Set 3		Set 4		Set 5	
		Reps	Weight	Reps	Weight	Reps	Weight	Reps	Weight	Reps	Weight
Group 1											
Group 2											
Group 3											
Group 4											
Abs											

Cardio

Cardio Activity:

Average Heart Rate:

Duration:

Notes:

START TIME:_____   END TIME:_____

DATE:_____

Daily Nutrition Journal   Week ⚪   Day ⚪

	Food	Serving Size	Calories	Carbs (grams)	Protein (grams)	Fat (grams)
Meal 1						
Meal 2						
Meal 3						
Meal 4						
Meal 5						
Meal 6						
Total						

DATE:_____

Daily Workout Journal   Week ⬤   Day ⬤

Exercise	Rest	Set 1 Reps	Set 1 Weight	Set 2 Reps	Set 2 Weight	Set 3 Reps	Set 3 Weight	Set 4 Reps	Set 4 Weight	Set 5 Reps	Set 5 Weight
Group 1											
Group 2											
Group 3											
Group 4											
Abs											

Cardio

Cardio Activity: Notes:

Average Heart Rate:

Duration:

START TIME:_____   **END TIME:**_____

DATE:_____

Daily Nutrition Journal   Week ⬤   Day ⬤

	Food	Serving Size	Calories	Carbs (grams)	Protein (grams)	Fat (grams)
Meal 1						
Meal 2						
Meal 3						
Meal 4						
Meal 5						
Meal 6						
Total						

DATE:_____

Daily Workout Journal

Week ⚪ Day ⚪

	Exercise	Rest	Set 1 Reps	Set 1 Weight	Set 2 Reps	Set 2 Weight	Set 3 Reps	Set 3 Weight	Set 4 Reps	Set 4 Weight	Set 5 Reps	Set 5 Weight	
Group 1													**Group 1**
Group 2													**Group 2**
Group 3													**Group 3**
Group 4													**Group 4**
Abs													**Abs**

Cardio	Cardio Activity:	Notes:	**Notes**
	Average Heart Rate:		
	Duration:		

START TIME:_____   END TIME:_____

DATE:_____

Daily Nutrition Journal

Week ⬤ Day ⬤

	Food	Serving Size	Calories	Carbs (grams)	Protein (grams)	Fat (grams)
Meal 1						
Meal 2						
Meal 3						
Meal 4						
Meal 5						
Meal 6						
Total						

DATE:_____

Daily Workout Journal Week ◯ Day ◯

Exercise	Rest	Set 1 Reps	Weight	Set 2 Reps	Weight	Set 3 Reps	Weight	Set 4 Reps	Weight	Set 5 Reps	Weight
Group 1											
Group 2											
Group 3											
Group 4											
Abs											

Cardio Activity: Notes:

Average Heart Rate:

Duration:

START TIME:_____   **END TIME:**_____

DATE:_____

Daily Nutrition Journal

Week ◯　Day ◯

	Food	Serving Size	Calories	Carbs (grams)	Protein (grams)	Fat (grams)
Meal 1						
Meal 2						
Meal 3						
Meal 4						
Meal 5						
Meal 6						
Total						

DATE:_____

Daily Workout Journal

Week ⬤ Day ⬤

	Exercise	Rest	Set 1 Reps	Weight	Set 2 Reps	Weight	Set 3 Reps	Weight	Set 4 Reps	Weight	Set 5 Reps	Weight	
Group 1													**Group 1**
Group 2													**Group 2**
Group 3													**Group 3**
Group 4													**Group 4**
Abs													**Abs**

Cardio	Cardio Activity:	Notes:	**Notes**
	Average Heart Rate:		
	Duration:		

START TIME:_____   END TIME:_____

DATE:_____

Daily Nutrition Journal

Week ◯ Day ◯

	Food	Serving Size	Calories	Carbs (grams)	Protein (grams)	Fat (grams)
Meal 1						
Meal 2						
Meal 3						
Meal 4						
Meal 5						
Meal 6						
Total						

DATE:_____

Daily Workout Journal

Week ⬤   Day ⬤

Exercise	Rest	Set 1		Set 2		Set 3		Set 4		Set 5	
		Reps	Weight	Reps	Weight	Reps	Weight	Reps	Weight	Reps	Weight
Group 1											
Group 2											
Group 3											
Group 4											
Abs											

Cardio

Cardio Activity: Notes:

Average Heart Rate:

Duration:

Notes

START TIME:_____   END TIME:_____

DATE:_____

Daily Nutrition Journal

Week ●   Day ●

	Food	Serving Size	Calories	Carbs (grams)	Protein (grams)	Fat (grams)
Meal 1						
Meal 2						
Meal 3						
Meal 4						
Meal 5						
Meal 6						
Total						

DATE:_____

Daily Workout Journal

Week ⚪   Day ⚪

	Exercise	Rest	Set 1 Reps	Weight	Set 2 Reps	Weight	Set 3 Reps	Weight	Set 4 Reps	Weight	Set 5 Reps	Weight	
Group 1													**Group 1**
Group 2													**Group 2**
Group 3													**Group 3**
Group 4													**Group 4**
Abs													**Abs**

Cardio	Cardio Activity: Notes: Average Heart Rate: Duration:	**Notes**

START TIME:_____   END TIME:_____

DATE:_____

Daily Nutrition Journal   Week ◯   Day ◯

	Food	Serving Size	Calories	Carbs (grams)	Protein (grams)	Fat (grams)
Meal 1						
Meal 2						
Meal 3						
Meal 4						
Meal 5						
Meal 6						
Total						

DATE:_____

Daily Workout Journal

Week ◯   Day ◯

	Exercise	Rest	Set 1 Reps	Weight	Set 2 Reps	Weight	Set 3 Reps	Weight	Set 4 Reps	Weight	Set 5 Reps	Weight	
Group 1													**Group 1**
Group 2													**Group 2**
Group 3													**Group 3**
Group 4													**Group 4**
Abs													**Abs**

Cardio	Cardio Activity: Average Heart Rate: Duration:	Notes:	**Notes**

START TIME:_____   **END TIME:**_____

DATE:_____

Daily Nutrition Journal

Week ⬤   Day ⬤

	Food	Serving Size	Calories	Carbs (grams)	Protein (grams)	Fat (grams)
Meal 1						
Meal 2						
Meal 3						
Meal 4						
Meal 5						
Meal 6						
Total						

DATE:_____

Daily Workout Journal   Week ⬤   Day ⬤

Exercise	Rest	Set 1 Reps	Set 1 Weight	Set 2 Reps	Set 2 Weight	Set 3 Reps	Set 3 Weight	Set 4 Reps	Set 4 Weight	Set 5 Reps	Set 5 Weight
Group 1											
Group 2											
Group 3											
Group 4											
Abs											

Cardio

Cardio Activity: Notes:

Average Heart Rate:

Duration:

START TIME:_____   **END TIME:**_____

DATE:_____

Daily Nutrition Journal

Week ⬤   Day ⬤

	Food	Serving Size	Calories	Carbs (grams)	Protein (grams)	Fat (grams)
Meal 1						
Meal 2						
Meal 3						
Meal 4						
Meal 5						
Meal 6						
Total						

DATE:_____

Daily Workout Journal

Week ⚪ Day ⚪

Exercise	Rest	Set 1		Set 2		Set 3		Set 4		Set 5	
		Reps	Weight	Reps	Weight	Reps	Weight	Reps	Weight	Reps	Weight
Group 1											
Group 2											
Group 3											
Group 4											
Abs											

Cardio

Cardio Activity:

Average Heart Rate:

Duration:

Notes:

START TIME:_____   **END TIME:**_____

DATE:_____

Daily Nutrition Journal   Week ●   Day ●

	Food	Serving Size	Calories	Carbs (grams)	Protein (grams)	Fat (grams)
Meal 1						
Meal 2						
Meal 3						
Meal 4						
Meal 5						
Meal 6						
Total						

DATE:_____

Daily Workout Journal   Week ⬤   Day ⬤

	Exercise	Rest	Set 1 Reps	Weight	Set 2 Reps	Weight	Set 3 Reps	Weight	Set 4 Reps	Weight	Set 5 Reps	Weight	
Group 1													Group 1
Group 2													Group 2
Group 3													Group 3
Group 4													Group 4
Abs													Abs

Cardio	Cardio Activity: Average Heart Rate: Duration:	Notes:	Notes

START TIME:_____   **END TIME:**_____

DATE:_____

Daily Nutrition Journal   Week ⬤   Day ⬤

	Food	Serving Size	Calories	Carbs (grams)	Protein (grams)	Fat (grams)
Meal 1						
Meal 2						
Meal 3						
Meal 4						
Meal 5						
Meal 6						
Total						

DATE:_____

Daily Workout Journal   Week ⬤   Day ⬤

	Exercise	Rest	Set 1 Reps	Weight	Set 2 Reps	Weight	Set 3 Reps	Weight	Set 4 Reps	Weight	Set 5 Reps	Weight
Group 1												
Group 2												
Group 3												
Group 4												
Abs												

Cardio

Cardio Activity: Notes:

Average Heart Rate:

Duration:

START TIME:_____   **END TIME:**_____

DATE:_____

Daily Nutrition Journal

Week ● Day ●

	Food	Serving Size	Calories	Carbs (grams)	Protein (grams)	Fat (grams)
Meal 1						
Meal 2						
Meal 3						
Meal 4						
Meal 5						
Meal 6						
Total						

DATE:_____

Daily Workout Journal

Week ⬤   Day ⬤

Exercise	Rest	Set 1		Set 2		Set 3		Set 4		Set 5	
		Reps	Weight	Reps	Weight	Reps	Weight	Reps	Weight	Reps	Weight
Group 1											
Group 2											
Group 3											
Group 4											
Abs											

Cardio

Cardio Activity: Notes:

Average Heart Rate:

Duration:

Notes

START TIME:_____   END TIME:_____

DATE:_____

Daily Nutrition Journal   Week ⬤   Day ⬤

	Food	Serving Size	Calories	Carbs (grams)	Protein (grams)	Fat (grams)
Meal 1						
Meal 2						
Meal 3						
Meal 4						
Meal 5						
Meal 6						
Total						

DATE:_____

Daily Workout Journal

Week ● Day ●

	Exercise	Rest	Set 1 Reps	Weight	Set 2 Reps	Weight	Set 3 Reps	Weight	Set 4 Reps	Weight	Set 5 Reps	Weight	
Group 1													**Group 1**
Group 2													**Group 2**
Group 3													**Group 3**
Group 4													**Group 4**
Abs													**Abs**

Cardio

Cardio Activity: Notes:
Average Heart Rate:
Duration:

Notes

START TIME:_____   END TIME:_____

DATE:_____

Daily Nutrition Journal   Week ⬤   Day ⬤

	Food	Serving Size	Calories	Carbs (grams)	Protein (grams)	Fat (grams)
Meal 1						
Meal 2						
Meal 3						
Meal 4						
Meal 5						
Meal 6						
Total						

DATE:_____

	Exercise	Rest	Set 1 Reps	Set 1 Weight	Set 2 Reps	Set 2 Weight	Set 3 Reps	Set 3 Weight	Set 4 Reps	Set 4 Weight	Set 5 Reps	Set 5 Weight	
Daily Workout Journal									Week ●		Day ●		
Group 1													Group 1
Group 2													Group 2
Group 3													Group 3
Group 4													Group 4
Abs													Abs
Cardio	Cardio Activity: Average Heart Rate: Duration:				Notes:								Notes

START TIME:_____   **END TIME:**_____

DATE:_____

Daily Nutrition Journal

Week ⚪ Day ⚪

	Food	Serving Size	Calories	Carbs (grams)	Protein (grams)	Fat (grams)
Meal 1						
Meal 2						
Meal 3						
Meal 4						
Meal 5						
Meal 6						
Total						

DATE:_____

Daily Workout Journal   Week ⬤   Day ⬤

	Exercise	Rest	Set 1 Reps	Weight	Set 2 Reps	Weight	Set 3 Reps	Weight	Set 4 Reps	Weight	Set 5 Reps	Weight
Group 1												
Group 2												
Group 3												
Group 4												
Abs												

Cardio
Cardio Activity: Notes:
Average Heart Rate:
Duration:

START TIME:_____   **END TIME:**_____

DATE:_____

Daily Nutrition Journal   Week ⬤   Day ⬤

	Food	Serving Size	Calories	Carbs (grams)	Protein (grams)	Fat (grams)
Meal 1						
Meal 2						
Meal 3						
Meal 4						
Meal 5						
Meal 6						
Total						

DATE:_____

Daily Workout Journal

Week ◯ Day ◯

	Exercise	Rest	Set 1 Reps	Set 1 Weight	Set 2 Reps	Set 2 Weight	Set 3 Reps	Set 3 Weight	Set 4 Reps	Set 4 Weight	Set 5 Reps	Set 5 Weight	
Group 1													**Group 1**
Group 2													**Group 2**
Group 3													**Group 3**
Group 4													**Group 4**
Abs													**Abs**
Cardio	Cardio Activity: Average Heart Rate: Duration:				Notes:								**Notes**

START TIME:_____   **END TIME:**_____

DATE:_____

Daily Nutrition Journal   Week ●   Day ●

	Food	Serving Size	Calories	Carbs (grams)	Protein (grams)	Fat (grams)
Meal 1						
Meal 2						
Meal 3						
Meal 4						
Meal 5						
Meal 6						
Total						

DATE:_____

Daily Workout Journal

Week ⬤   Day ⬤

	Exercise	Rest	Set 1 Reps	Weight	Set 2 Reps	Weight	Set 3 Reps	Weight	Set 4 Reps	Weight	Set 5 Reps	Weight	
Group 1													**Group 1**
Group 2													**Group 2**
Group 3													**Group 3**
Group 4													**Group 4**
Abs													**Abs**
Cardio	Cardio Activity: Average Heart Rate: Duration:		Notes:										**Notes**

START TIME:_____   **END TIME:**_____

DATE:_____

Daily Nutrition Journal Week ⬤ Day ⬤

	Food	Serving Size	Calories	Carbs (grams)	Protein (grams)	Fat (grams)
Meal 1						
Meal 2						
Meal 3						
Meal 4						
Meal 5						
Meal 6						
Total						

DATE:_____

Daily Workout Journal

Week ⬤ Day ⬤

	Exercise	Rest	Set 1 Reps	Set 1 Weight	Set 2 Reps	Set 2 Weight	Set 3 Reps	Set 3 Weight	Set 4 Reps	Set 4 Weight	Set 5 Reps	Set 5 Weight
Group 1												
Group 2												
Group 3												
Group 4												
Abs												

Cardio Activity:

Average Heart Rate:

Duration:

Notes:

START TIME:_____   END TIME:_____

DATE:_____

Daily Nutrition Journal

Week ◯   Day ◯

	Food	Serving Size	Calories	Carbs (grams)	Protein (grams)	Fat (grams)
Meal 1						
Meal 2						
Meal 3						
Meal 4						
Meal 5						
Meal 6						
Total						

DATE:_____

Daily Workout Journal

Week ⬤ Day ⬤

	Exercise	Rest	Set 1 Reps	Weight	Set 2 Reps	Weight	Set 3 Reps	Weight	Set 4 Reps	Weight	Set 5 Reps	Weight
Group 1												
Group 2												
Group 3												
Group 4												
Abs												

Cardio

Cardio Activity: Notes:

Average Heart Rate:

Duration:

START TIME:_____   END TIME:_____

DATE:_____

Daily Nutrition Journal   Week ●   Day ●

	Food	Serving Size	Calories	Carbs (grams)	Protein (grams)	Fat (grams)
Meal 1						
Meal 2						
Meal 3						
Meal 4						
Meal 5						
Meal 6						
Total						

DATE:_____

Daily Workout Journal

Week ⚪ Day ⚪

	Exercise	Rest	Set 1 Reps	Weight	Set 2 Reps	Weight	Set 3 Reps	Weight	Set 4 Reps	Weight	Set 5 Reps	Weight	
Group 1													**Group 1**
Group 2													**Group 2**
Group 3													**Group 3**
Group 4													**Group 4**
Abs													**Abs**

Cardio	Cardio Activity:	Notes:	**Notes**
	Average Heart Rate:		
	Duration:		

START TIME:_____   END TIME:_____

DATE:_____

Daily Nutrition Journal   Week ⬤   Day ⬤

	Food	Serving Size	Calories	Carbs (grams)	Protein (grams)	Fat (grams)	
Meal 1							**Meal 1**
Meal 2							**Meal 2**
Meal 3							**Meal 3**
Meal 4							**Meal 4**
Meal 5							**Meal 5**
Meal 6							**Meal 6**
Total							

DATE:_____

Daily Workout Journal

Week ⬤   Day ⬤

	Exercise	Rest	Set 1 Reps	Weight	Set 2 Reps	Weight	Set 3 Reps	Weight	Set 4 Reps	Weight	Set 5 Reps	Weight	
Group 1													**Group 1**
Group 2													**Group 2**
Group 3													**Group 3**
Group 4													**Group 4**
Abs													**Abs**
Cardio	Cardio Activity: Average Heart Rate: Duration:			Notes:									**Notes**

START TIME:_____   **END TIME:**_____

DATE:_____

Daily Nutrition Journal Week ⬤ Day ⬤

	Food	Serving Size	Calories	Carbs (grams)	Protein (grams)	Fat (grams)
Meal 1						
Meal 2						
Meal 3						
Meal 4						
Meal 5						
Meal 6						
Total						

DATE:_____

Daily Workout Journal

Week ⬤ Day ⬤

	Exercise	Rest	Set 1 Reps	Set 1 Weight	Set 2 Reps	Set 2 Weight	Set 3 Reps	Set 3 Weight	Set 4 Reps	Set 4 Weight	Set 5 Reps	Set 5 Weight	
Group 1													**Group 1**
Group 2													**Group 2**
Group 3													**Group 3**
Group 4													**Group 4**
Abs													**Abs**

Cardio

Cardio Activity: Notes:

Average Heart Rate:

Duration:

Notes

START TIME:_____   **END TIME:**_____

DATE:_____

Daily Nutrition Journal   Week ⬤   Day ⬤

	Food	Serving Size	Calories	Carbs (grams)	Protein (grams)	Fat (grams)
Meal 1						
Meal 2						
Meal 3						
Meal 4						
Meal 5						
Meal 6						
Total						

DATE:_____

Daily Workout Journal   Week ⬤   Day ⬤

	Exercise	Rest	Set 1		Set 2		Set 3		Set 4		Set 5	
			Reps	Weight	Reps	Weight	Reps	Weight	Reps	Weight	Reps	Weight
Group 1												
Group 2												
Group 3												
Group 4												
Abs												

Cardio	Cardio Activity:	Notes:	**Notes**
	Average Heart Rate:		
	Duration:		

START TIME:_____   **END TIME:**_____

DATE: _____

Daily Nutrition Journal

Week ⬤ Day ⬤

	Food	Serving Size	Calories	Carbs (grams)	Protein (grams)	Fat (grams)
Meal 1						
Meal 2						
Meal 3						
Meal 4						
Meal 5						
Meal 6						
Total						

DATE:_____

Daily Workout Journal

Week ◯ Day ◯

Exercise	Rest	Set 1 Reps	Weight	Set 2 Reps	Weight	Set 3 Reps	Weight	Set 4 Reps	Weight	Set 5 Reps	Weight
Group 1											
Group 2											
Group 3											
Group 4											
Abs											

Cardio

Cardio Activity: Notes:

Average Heart Rate:

Duration:

START TIME:_____   **END TIME:**_____

DATE:_____

Daily Nutrition Journal

	Food	Serving Size	Calories	Carbs (grams)	Protein (grams)	Fat (grams)
Meal 1						
Meal 2						
Meal 3						
Meal 4						
Meal 5						
Meal 6						
Total						

DATE:_____

Daily Workout Journal

Week ⬤   Day ⬤

	Exercise	Rest	Set 1 Reps	Weight	Set 2 Reps	Weight	Set 3 Reps	Weight	Set 4 Reps	Weight	Set 5 Reps	Weight
Group 1												
Group 2												
Group 3												
Group 4												
Abs												

Cardio	Cardio Activity: Notes:	**Notes**
	Average Heart Rate:	
	Duration:	

START TIME:_____   END TIME:_____

DATE:_____

Daily Nutrition Journal   Week ⬤   Day ⬤

	Food	Serving Size	Calories	Carbs (grams)	Protein (grams)	Fat (grams)
Meal 1						
Meal 2						
Meal 3						
Meal 4						
Meal 5						
Meal 6						
Total						

DATE:_____

Daily Workout Journal

Week ⬤   Day ⬤

	Exercise	Rest	Set 1		Set 2		Set 3		Set 4		Set 5	
			Reps	Weight	Reps	Weight	Reps	Weight	Reps	Weight	Reps	Weight
Group 1												
Group 2												
Group 3												
Group 4												
Abs												
Cardio	Cardio Activity: Average Heart Rate: Duration:			Notes:								**Notes**

START TIME:_____   END TIME:_____

DATE:_____

Daily Nutrition Journal Week ⬤ Day ⬤

	Food	Serving Size	Calories	Carbs (grams)	Protein (grams)	Fat (grams)
Meal 1						
Meal 2						
Meal 3						
Meal 4						
Meal 5						
Meal 6						
Total						

DATE:_____

Daily Workout Journal

Week ⚪ Day ⚪

	Exercise	Rest	Set 1 Reps	Set 1 Weight	Set 2 Reps	Set 2 Weight	Set 3 Reps	Set 3 Weight	Set 4 Reps	Set 4 Weight	Set 5 Reps	Set 5 Weight	
Group 1													Group 1
Group 2													Group 2
Group 3													Group 3
Group 4													Group 4
Abs													Abs

Cardio

Cardio Activity: Notes:

Average Heart Rate:

Duration:

Notes

START TIME:_____   END TIME:_____

DATE:_____

Daily Nutrition Journal   Week ●   Day ●

	Food	Serving Size	Calories	Carbs (grams)	Protein (grams)	Fat (grams)
Meal 1						
Meal 2						
Meal 3						
Meal 4						
Meal 5						
Meal 6						
Total						

DATE:_____

Daily Workout Journal   Week ⚪   Day ⚪

Exercise	Rest	Set 1 Reps	Weight	Set 2 Reps	Weight	Set 3 Reps	Weight	Set 4 Reps	Weight	Set 5 Reps	Weight
Group 1											
Group 2											
Group 3											
Group 4											
Abs											

Cardio

Cardio Activity: Notes:

Average Heart Rate:

Duration:

START TIME:_____   **END TIME:**_____

DATE:_____

Daily Nutrition Journal   Week ○   Day ○

	Food	Serving Size	Calories	Carbs (grams)	Protein (grams)	Fat (grams)
Meal 1						
Meal 2						
Meal 3						
Meal 4						
Meal 5						
Meal 6						
Total						

DATE:_____

Daily Workout Journal

Week ● Day ●

	Exercise	Rest	Set 1 Reps Weight		Set 2 Reps Weight		Set 3 Reps Weight		Set 4 Reps Weight		Set 5 Reps Weight		
Group 1													**Group 1**
Group 2													**Group 2**
Group 3													**Group 3**
Group 4													**Group 4**
Abs													**Abs**
Cardio	Cardio Activity: Average Heart Rate: Duration:		Notes:										**Notes**

START TIME:_____   **END TIME:**_____

DATE:_____

Daily Nutrition Journal

	Food	Serving Size	Calories	Carbs (grams)	Protein (grams)	Fat (grams)
Meal 1						
Meal 2						
Meal 3						
Meal 4						
Meal 5						
Meal 6						
Total						

DATE:_____

Daily Workout Journal — Week ⬤ Day ⬤

Exercise	Rest	Set 1 Reps	Set 1 Weight	Set 2 Reps	Set 2 Weight	Set 3 Reps	Set 3 Weight	Set 4 Reps	Set 4 Weight	Set 5 Reps	Set 5 Weight
Group 1											
Group 2											
Group 3											
Group 4											
Abs											

Cardio

Cardio Activity:

Average Heart Rate:

Duration:

Notes:

START TIME:_____   END TIME:_____

DATE:_____

Daily Nutrition Journal

Week ●   Day ●

	Food	Serving Size	Calories	Carbs (grams)	Protein (grams)	Fat (grams)
Meal 1						
Meal 2						
Meal 3						
Meal 4						
Meal 5						
Meal 6						
Total						

DATE:_____

Daily Workout Journal

Week ●   Day ●

	Exercise	Rest	Set 1 Reps	Weight	Set 2 Reps	Weight	Set 3 Reps	Weight	Set 4 Reps	Weight	Set 5 Reps	Weight
Group 1												
Group 2												
Group 3												
Group 4												
Abs												
Cardio	Cardio Activity:					Notes:						
	Average Heart Rate:											
	Duration:											

START TIME:_____   END TIME:_____

DATE:_____

Daily Nutrition Journal   Week ◯   Day ◯

	Food	Serving Size	Calories	Carbs (grams)	Protein (grams)	Fat (grams)
Meal 1						
Meal 2						
Meal 3						
Meal 4						
Meal 5						
Meal 6						
Total						

DATE:_____

Daily Workout Journal

Week ⬤   Day ⬤

Exercise	Rest	Set 1 Reps	Weight	Set 2 Reps	Weight	Set 3 Reps	Weight	Set 4 Reps	Weight	Set 5 Reps	Weight
Group 1											
Group 2											
Group 3											
Group 4											
Abs											

Cardio

Cardio Activity:

Average Heart Rate:

Duration:

Notes:

START TIME:_____　　　　END TIME:_____

DATE:_____

Daily Nutrition Journal

Week ⬤ Day ⬤

	Food	Serving Size	Calories	Carbs (grams)	Protein (grams)	Fat (grams)
Meal 1						
Meal 2						
Meal 3						
Meal 4						
Meal 5						
Meal 6						
Total						

DATE:_____

Daily Workout Journal   Week ⬤   Day ⬤

	Exercise	Rest	Set 1 Reps	Set 1 Weight	Set 2 Reps	Set 2 Weight	Set 3 Reps	Set 3 Weight	Set 4 Reps	Set 4 Weight	Set 5 Reps	Set 5 Weight
Group 1												
Group 2												
Group 3												
Group 4												
Abs												

Cardio

Cardio Activity: Notes:

Average Heart Rate:

Duration:

START TIME:_____   **END TIME:**_____

DATE: _____

Daily Nutrition Journal   Week ⬤   Day ⬤

	Food	Serving Size	Calories	Carbs (grams)	Protein (grams)	Fat (grams)
Meal 1						
Meal 2						
Meal 3						
Meal 4						
Meal 5						
Meal 6						
Total						

DATE:_____

Daily Workout Journal

Week ⬤ Day ⬤

	Exercise	Rest	Set 1 Reps	Set 1 Weight	Set 2 Reps	Set 2 Weight	Set 3 Reps	Set 3 Weight	Set 4 Reps	Set 4 Weight	Set 5 Reps	Set 5 Weight	
Group 1													Group 1
Group 2													Group 2
Group 3													Group 3
Group 4													Group 4
Abs													Abs
Cardio	Cardio Activity: Average Heart Rate: Duration:				Notes:								Notes

START TIME:_____   END TIME:_____

DATE:_____

Daily Nutrition Journal

Week ● Day ●

	Food	Serving Size	Calories	Carbs (grams)	Protein (grams)	Fat (grams)
Meal 1						
Meal 2						
Meal 3						
Meal 4						
Meal 5						
Meal 6						
Total						

DATE:_____

Daily Workout Journal   Week ⬤   Day ⬤

	Exercise	Rest	Set 1 Reps	Weight	Set 2 Reps	Weight	Set 3 Reps	Weight	Set 4 Reps	Weight	Set 5 Reps	Weight	
Group 1													**Group 1**
Group 2													**Group 2**
Group 3													**Group 3**
Group 4													**Group 4**
Abs													**Abs**

Cardio	Cardio Activity: Notes: Average Heart Rate: Duration:	**Notes**

START TIME:_____   **END TIME:**_____

DATE:_____

Daily Nutrition Journal

Week ● Day ●

	Food	Serving Size	Calories	Carbs (grams)	Protein (grams)	Fat (grams)
Meal 1						
Meal 2						
Meal 3						
Meal 4						
Meal 5						
Meal 6						
Total						

DATE:_____

Daily Workout Journal   Week ⬤   Day ⬤

	Exercise	Rest	Set 1 Reps	Weight	Set 2 Reps	Weight	Set 3 Reps	Weight	Set 4 Reps	Weight	Set 5 Reps	Weight	
Group 1													**Group 1**
Group 2													**Group 2**
Group 3													**Group 3**
Group 4													**Group 4**
Abs													**Abs**

Cardio

Cardio Activity: Notes:

Average Heart Rate:

Duration:

Notes

START TIME:_____   **END TIME:**_____

DATE:_____

Daily Nutrition Journal

Week ○ Day ○

	Food	Serving Size	Calories	Carbs (grams)	Protein (grams)	Fat (grams)
Meal 1						
Meal 2						
Meal 3						
Meal 4						
Meal 5						
Meal 6						
Total						

DATE:_____

Daily Workout Journal   Week ⬤   Day ⬤

Exercise	Rest	Set 1		Set 2		Set 3		Set 4		Set 5	
		Reps	Weight	Reps	Weight	Reps	Weight	Reps	Weight	Reps	Weight
Group 1											
Group 2											
Group 3											
Group 4											
Abs											

Cardio

Cardio Activity: Notes:

Average Heart Rate:

Duration:

START TIME:_____   **END TIME:**_____

DATE:_____

Daily Nutrition Journal

Week ⬤ Day ⬤

	Food	Serving Size	Calories	Carbs (grams)	Protein (grams)	Fat (grams)
Meal 1						
Meal 2						
Meal 3						
Meal 4						
Meal 5						
Meal 6						
Total						

DATE:_____

Daily Workout Journal

Week ●   Day ●

	Exercise	Rest	Set 1		Set 2		Set 3		Set 4		Set 5	
			Reps	Weight	Reps	Weight	Reps	Weight	Reps	Weight	Reps	Weight
Group 1												
Group 2												
Group 3												
Group 4												
Abs												

Cardio	Cardio Activity:	Notes:	**Notes**
	Average Heart Rate:		
	Duration:		

START TIME:_____   **END TIME:**_____

DATE:_____

Daily Nutrition Journal

Week ⚪ Day ⚪

	Food	Serving Size	Calories	Carbs (grams)	Protein (grams)	Fat (grams)
Meal 1						
Meal 2						
Meal 3						
Meal 4						
Meal 5						
Meal 6						
Total						

DATE:_____

Daily Workout Journal   Week ◯   Day ◯

Exercise	Rest	Set 1 Reps	Set 1 Weight	Set 2 Reps	Set 2 Weight	Set 3 Reps	Set 3 Weight	Set 4 Reps	Set 4 Weight	Set 5 Reps	Set 5 Weight
Group 1											
Group 2											
Group 3											
Group 4											
Abs											

Cardio
Cardio Activity:
Average Heart Rate:
Duration:

Notes:

START TIME:_____   END TIME:_____

DATE:_____

Daily Nutrition Journal   Week ⬤   Day ⬤

	Food	Serving Size	Calories	Carbs (grams)	Protein (grams)	Fat (grams)
Meal 1						
Meal 2						
Meal 3						
Meal 4						
Meal 5						
Meal 6						
Total						

DATE:_____

Daily Workout Journal

Week ⬤ Day ⬤

	Exercise	Rest	Set 1 Reps	Set 1 Weight	Set 2 Reps	Set 2 Weight	Set 3 Reps	Set 3 Weight	Set 4 Reps	Set 4 Weight	Set 5 Reps	Set 5 Weight	
Group 1													**Group 1**
Group 2													**Group 2**
Group 3													**Group 3**
Group 4													**Group 4**
Abs													**Abs**

Cardio	Cardio Activity:	Notes:	**Notes**
	Average Heart Rate:		
	Duration:		

START TIME:_____   END TIME:_____

DATE:_____

Daily Nutrition Journal   Week ⬤   Day ⬤

	Food	Serving Size	Calories	Carbs (grams)	Protein (grams)	Fat (grams)
Meal 1						
Meal 2						
Meal 3						
Meal 4						
Meal 5						
Meal 6						
Total						

DATE:_____

Daily Workout Journal   Week ⚪   Day ⚪

	Exercise	Rest	Set 1		Set 2		Set 3		Set 4		Set 5	
			Reps	Weight	Reps	Weight	Reps	Weight	Reps	Weight	Reps	Weight
Group 1												
Group 2												
Group 3												
Group 4												
Abs												

Cardio

Cardio Activity: Notes:

Average Heart Rate:

Duration:

START TIME:_____   END TIME:_____

DATE:_____

Daily Nutrition Journal   Week ⬤   Day ⬤

	Food	Serving Size	Calories	Carbs (grams)	Protein (grams)	Fat (grams)
Meal 1						
Meal 2						
Meal 3						
Meal 4						
Meal 5						
Meal 6						
Total						

DATE:_____

Daily Workout Journal

Week ⬤ Day ⬤

	Exercise	Rest	Set 1		Set 2		Set 3		Set 4		Set 5	
			Reps	Weight	Reps	Weight	Reps	Weight	Reps	Weight	Reps	Weight
Group 1												
Group 2												
Group 3												
Group 4												
Abs												

Cardio | Cardio Activity: | | Notes: | | **Notes**
Average Heart Rate:
Duration:

START TIME:_____   END TIME:_____

DATE:_____

Daily Nutrition Journal

Week ◯ Day ◯

	Food	Serving Size	Calories	Carbs (grams)	Protein (grams)	Fat (grams)
Meal 1						
Meal 2						
Meal 3						
Meal 4						
Meal 5						
Meal 6						
Total						

DATE:_____

Daily Workout Journal

Week ⚪ Day ⚪

Exercise	Rest	Set 1		Set 2		Set 3		Set 4		Set 5	
		Reps	Weight	Reps	Weight	Reps	Weight	Reps	Weight	Reps	Weight
Group 1											
Group 2											
Group 3											
Group 4											
Abs											

Cardio

Cardio Activity: Notes:

Average Heart Rate:

Duration:

START TIME:_____   **END TIME:**_____

DATE:_____

Daily Nutrition Journal   Week ⬤   Day ⬤

	Food	Serving Size	Calories	Carbs (grams)	Protein (grams)	Fat (grams)
Meal 1						
Meal 2						
Meal 3						
Meal 4						
Meal 5						
Meal 6						
Total						

DATE:_____

Daily Workout Journal Week ● Day ●

Exercise	Rest	Set 1 Reps	Weight	Set 2 Reps	Weight	Set 3 Reps	Weight	Set 4 Reps	Weight	Set 5 Reps	Weight
Group 1											
Group 2											
Group 3											
Group 4											
Abs											

Cardio

Cardio Activity: Notes:

Average Heart Rate:

Duration:

START TIME:_____   END TIME:_____

DATE:_____

Daily Nutrition Journal

Week ⬤ Day ⬤

	Food	Serving Size	Calories	Carbs (grams)	Protein (grams)	Fat (grams)
Meal 1						
Meal 2						
Meal 3						
Meal 4						
Meal 5						
Meal 6						
Total						

DATE:_____

Daily Workout Journal

Week ⬤ Day ⬤

	Exercise	Rest	Set 1		Set 2		Set 3		Set 4		Set 5	
			Reps	Weight	Reps	Weight	Reps	Weight	Reps	Weight	Reps	Weight
Group 1												
Group 2												
Group 3												
Group 4												
Abs												

Cardio		Notes
Cardio Activity:	Notes:	
Average Heart Rate:		
Duration:		

START TIME:_____ END TIME:_____

DATE:_____

Daily Nutrition Journal

Week ●   Day ●

	Food	Serving Size	Calories	Carbs (grams)	Protein (grams)	Fat (grams)
Meal 1						
Meal 2						
Meal 3						
Meal 4						
Meal 5						
Meal 6						
Total						

DATE:_____

Daily Workout Journal

Week ⬤   Day ⬤

Exercise	Rest	Set 1		Set 2		Set 3		Set 4		Set 5	
		Reps	Weight	Reps	Weight	Reps	Weight	Reps	Weight	Reps	Weight
Group 1											
Group 2											
Group 3											
Group 4											
Abs											

Cardio

Cardio Activity: Notes:

Average Heart Rate:

Duration:

START TIME:_____   **END TIME:**_____

DATE:_____

Daily Nutrition Journal   Week ⬤   Day ⬤

	Food	Serving Size	Calories	Carbs (grams)	Protein (grams)	Fat (grams)
Meal 1						
Meal 2						
Meal 3						
Meal 4						
Meal 5						
Meal 6						
Total						

DATE:_____

Daily Workout Journal   Week ○   Day ○

	Exercise	Rest	Set 1 Reps	Set 1 Weight	Set 2 Reps	Set 2 Weight	Set 3 Reps	Set 3 Weight	Set 4 Reps	Set 4 Weight	Set 5 Reps	Set 5 Weight	
Group 1													Group 1
Group 2													Group 2
Group 3													Group 3
Group 4													Group 4
Abs													Abs

Cardio	Cardio Activity: Notes:	Notes
	Average Heart Rate:	
	Duration:	

START TIME:_____   **END TIME:**_____

DATE:_____

Daily Nutrition Journal   Week ⬤   Day ⬤

	Food	Serving Size	Calories	Carbs (grams)	Protein (grams)	Fat (grams)
Meal 1						
Meal 2						
Meal 3						
Meal 4						
Meal 5						
Meal 6						
Total						

DATE:_____

Daily Workout Journal   Week ⚪   Day ⚪

Exercise	Rest	Set 1		Set 2		Set 3		Set 4		Set 5	
		Reps	Weight	Reps	Weight	Reps	Weight	Reps	Weight	Reps	Weight
Group 1											
Group 2											
Group 3											
Group 4											
Abs											

Cardio

Cardio Activity: Notes:

Average Heart Rate:

Duration:

START TIME:_____   **END TIME:**_____

DATE:_____

Daily Nutrition Journal   Week ○   Day ○

	Food	Serving Size	Calories	Carbs (grams)	Protein (grams)	Fat (grams)	
Meal 1							**Meal 1**
Meal 2							**Meal 2**
Meal 3							**Meal 3**
Meal 4							**Meal 4**
Meal 5							**Meal 5**
Meal 6							**Meal 6**
	Total						

DATE:_____

Daily Workout Journal Week ⬤ Day ⬤

Exercise	Rest	Set 1 Reps	Set 1 Weight	Set 2 Reps	Set 2 Weight	Set 3 Reps	Set 3 Weight	Set 4 Reps	Set 4 Weight	Set 5 Reps	Set 5 Weight
Group 1											
Group 2											
Group 3											
Group 4											
Abs											

Cardio

Cardio Activity: Notes:

Average Heart Rate:

Duration:

START TIME:_____ END TIME:_____

DATE:_____

Daily Nutrition Journal   Week ●   Day ●

	Food	Serving Size	Calories	Carbs (grams)	Protein (grams)	Fat (grams)
Meal 1						
Meal 2						
Meal 3						
Meal 4						
Meal 5						
Meal 6						
Total						

DATE:_____

Daily Workout Journal   Week ⬤   Day ⬤

	Exercise	Rest	Set 1 Reps	Set 1 Weight	Set 2 Reps	Set 2 Weight	Set 3 Reps	Set 3 Weight	Set 4 Reps	Set 4 Weight	Set 5 Reps	Set 5 Weight	
Group 1													Group 1
Group 2													Group 2
Group 3													Group 3
Group 4													Group 4
Abs													Abs

Cardio

Cardio Activity: Notes:

Average Heart Rate:

Duration:

Notes

START TIME:_____   END TIME:_____

DATE:_____

Daily Nutrition Journal

Week ⬤ Day ⬤

	Food	Serving Size	Calories	Carbs (grams)	Protein (grams)	Fat (grams)
Meal 1						
Meal 2						
Meal 3						
Meal 4						
Meal 5						
Meal 6						
Total						

DATE:_____

Daily Workout Journal   Week ⬤   Day ⬤

	Exercise	Rest	Set 1 Reps	Weight	Set 2 Reps	Weight	Set 3 Reps	Weight	Set 4 Reps	Weight	Set 5 Reps	Weight	
Group 1													**Group 1**
Group 2													**Group 2**
Group 3													**Group 3**
Group 4													**Group 4**
Abs													**Abs**
Cardio	Cardio Activity: Average Heart Rate: Duration:		Notes:										**Notes**

START TIME:_____   END TIME:_____

DATE:_____

Daily Nutrition Journal   Week ●   Day ●

	Food	Serving Size	Calories	Carbs (grams)	Protein (grams)	Fat (grams)
Meal 1						
Meal 2						
Meal 3						
Meal 4						
Meal 5						
Meal 6						
Total						

DATE:_____

Daily Workout Journal

Week ●   Day ●

Exercise	Rest	Set 1		Set 2		Set 3		Set 4		Set 5	
		Reps	Weight	Reps	Weight	Reps	Weight	Reps	Weight	Reps	Weight

Group 1

Group 2

Group 3

Group 4

Abs

Cardio

Cardio Activity: Notes:

Average Heart Rate:

Duration:

Notes

START TIME:_____   **END TIME:**_____

DATE:_____

Daily Nutrition Journal

Week ⬤   Day ⬤

	Food	Serving Size	Calories	Carbs (grams)	Protein (grams)	Fat (grams)
Meal 1						
Meal 2						
Meal 3						
Meal 4						
Meal 5						
Meal 6						
Total						

DATE:_____

Daily Workout Journal

Week ⬤ Day ⬤

	Exercise	Rest	Set 1		Set 2		Set 3		Set 4		Set 5	
			Reps	Weight	Reps	Weight	Reps	Weight	Reps	Weight	Reps	Weight
Group 1												
Group 2												
Group 3												
Group 4												
Abs												

Cardio		**Notes**
Cardio Activity:	Notes:	
Average Heart Rate:		
Duration:		

START TIME:_____   END TIME:_____

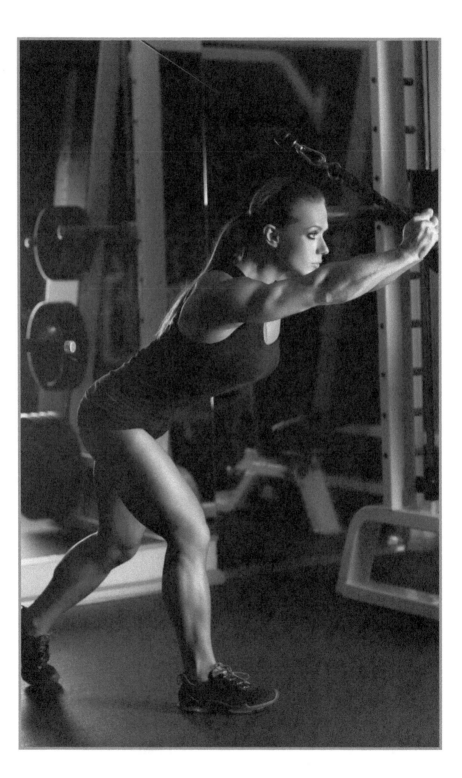

Next Steps for
Continued Results

After you finish 6 weeks of one of the Body Sculpting workouts in the previous section, assess your original goals and measure how far you have come. Then make new goals and select your next six-week workout!

ORIGINAL 6-WEEK GOALS

Lose _____ pounds of fat
Gain _____ pounds of muscle
Weigh _____ pounds

Have Measurements of:
Chest _____
Arms _____
Thighs _____
Calves _____
Waist _____
Hips _____

6-WEEK ACHIEVEMENTS

Lost _____ pounds of fat
Gained _____ pounds of muscle
Weigh _____ pounds

Measurements:
Chest _____ Gained _____ inches
Arms _____ Gained _____ inches
Thighs _____ Gained _____ inches
Calves _____ Gained _____ inches
Waist _____ Gained/Lost _____ inches
Hips _____ Gained/Lost _____ inches

ASSESSMENT

Did you achieve your goals?
If not, then answer the following questions:
- Were your goals realistic?

- Did you follow the training plan as laid out and adhere to the recom-

NEXT STEPS FOR CONTINUED RESULTS

mended repetitions, exercises, and rest periods? Could you have done something better?

- Did you follow the nutrition plan? Were you skipping meals? Did you drink alcohol during the weekends?
- Did you take your nutritional supplements?
- Did you sleep at least 7 hours each night?

Now look at the answers above and see what was missing in your program. When you set your new goals, make sure that whatever component was not followed 100% this time around, is followed the next time for better results.

Now that you have assessed how far you have come, be proud of your accomplishments, set new goals to get even better and select your next Body Sculpting Workout!

The biggest secrets to long-term success from a fitness program are to have the determination to stay consistent with your fitness program day in and day out for years to come, always setting new goals, and achieving higher levels of development.

TO CONTACT THE AUTHORS DIRECTLY, PLEASE VISIT:

WWW.HUGORIVERA.NET

WWW.JAMESVILLEPIGUE.COM

BE SURE TO VISIT OUR FACEBOOK PAGE
FOR FITNESS TIPS AND SUPPORT!

WWW.FACEBOOK.COM/BODYSCULPTINGBIBLES

GOT QUESTIONS?
NEED ANSWERS?
GO TO:

BODYSCULPTINGBIBLE.com
IT'S FITNESS 24/7

VIDEOS - WORKOUTS - FORUMS
ONLINE STORE

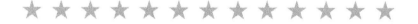